A Beginner's Guide to the Mediterranean Diet

Delicious, quick, and easy recipes

Justin A. Ryan

Contents

Chapter 1

Introduction

Dietary Guidelines for Americans (Dietary Guidelines for Americans)

The Mediterranean diet, which is one of the world's healthiest diets, has roots that date back to the days of Ancient Greece and Rome, despite the fact that this isn't a history lecture on the subject. Given the fact that these two civilizations were among the most successful on the planet, it should come as no surprise that the Mediterranean diet has endured as a result of its many health advantages.

It is crucial to highlight that, although the Mediterranean diet derives its name from the physical area in which it was developed, it was Greece and Italy who, since antiquity, were the two nations that actually brought it to life. These civilizations not only flourished and prospered where many others had failed, but - and many experts can corroborate this - they also ate exceedingly well, which was a contributing factor to their wealth.

Because of the temperature and geology of the area, there was not much space for a diet centered on the eating of red meat to emerge and flourish (meaning automatically reduced cholesterol levels). Although fish intake as an animal protein source was not widespread, there was a significant cultural tradition formed around it. During the ancient Greek period, fishing was one of the most important sources of revenue for the country's economy. The consumption of fish was thus significant. To mention a few, they often fished and consumed animals like sea bass, yellowfin tuna, and sprat.

Whole grains, fruits, vegetables, legumes, and olive oil, on the other hand, were also essential components of their nutritional intake. In this area, whole grains such as wheat and barley were particularly essential, since they were used to create bread and wine, among other things. Fruits and vegetables such as figs, cucumbers, artichokes, pears, and olives were utilized in daily cuisine - with certain items being kept for higher social strata and the preparation of feasts, festivities, and religious rites, while others were used for everyday cookery. In addition to beans and lentils, chickpeas and other legumes were often used in stews and other preparations. Then there's the fact that olive oil was regarded "liquid gold" by these people, who used it in their cooking and a variety of other activities throughout their lives. The fact that all of these foods were grown and traded locally made them indisputable foundational components for a Mediterranean diet that would ultimately define the whole region.

The use and trade of these foods were, in the end, the foundation of this society. However, it is probable that a combination of factors such as the Ancient Greek diet and socio-political condition as well as ancient Greek beliefs as well as location, trade, and other factors enabled the country to be the home to some of history's greatest thinkers and intellectuals. It wasn't long ago that even academics began to notice and research the importance of foods in a person's diet and general health. In fact, our line of thinking wasn't too far off the mark from reality. Food was first used as medicine by doctors in Ancient Greece, who prescribed certain meals and diets to heal a variety of diseases in both the body and the spirit. Not only did medical patients benefit from the meals that were often recommended, but so did the general public. In part due to the fact that the food was mostly from the region, everyone benefited in some manner from what is now known as the Mediterranean diet. Because of this nutritious diet, the citizens of both civilizations stood to gain significantly, and this benefit was reflected in their respective levels of wealth.

Throughout history, the diet has developed somewhat to include a few of additional items that are not necessarily native to the area, but the fundamental principles around which it was formed and structured have remained the same. The same can be said for one notion from their old medicine, which is still relevant today.

Generally speaking, in the presence of most illnesses, physicians examine the patient's food in addition to prescribing medicine. A partial, complete, temporary, or permanent modification of your current diet may be recommended if they believe it is deficient in specific nutrients or protein. There have been thousands of years since this event, yet the idea has not changed. Medicine, although being a scientific discipline, is unquestionably guided by a rather holistic perspective in its methods. In addition to assessing the patient's physical and mental health, as well as their overall lifestyle, including their food, physicians may propose dietary adjustments after the condition has been detected (although not always). Food is, and always will be, a kind of medicine for the body and the spirit in a variety of respects. In other words, it's critical to pay great attention to what you're eating and in what amounts at all times, particularly if you have one or more chronic ailments.

Accordingly, in the same way that the Ancient Greeks did, the Mediterranean diet seeks to create positive long-term changes in what you eat rather than in what amounts you consume. Many individuals from all around the globe have found the diet to be both intriguing and enticing because of this. The fact that there are no hard regulations means that it is not only healthful, but also like a blank canvas on which to paint. Consider it more of an eating pattern than a diet, one that you must get used to in order to achieve success. Following that, it will feel no different from the way you chose what to eat now (except that it will be far healthier). For the simple reason that, once again, the goal is not to count calories, but rather to become more aware of what you are eating.

The Mediterranean diet is so nutritious that it is beneficial to everyone, but it is particularly beneficial to those who want to lower their risk of cardiovascular disease and even avoid it. In this article, we will explain why the Mediterranean diet is regarded to be one of the healthiest diets in the world, with the assistance of fresh produce, seafood, legumes, whole grains, healthy fats, herbs, and a handful other healthier components. Prior to getting started on the food preparation, it is essential that you be aware of a few more considerations, so let's get started. A Guide to the Mediterranean Diet: What to Eat and What Not to Eat.

Essentially, the Mediterranean diet is intended to be as similar to the Ancient Greek diet as possible. However, this is not always the case. According to this way of thinking about it, you will be able to eat as if you were gods. While we cannot guarantee that you will acquire their abilities, one thing we can guarantee is that you will develop the capacity to fight against heart disease and other illnesses and disorders, among others.

The Mediterranean diet is not at all restricted, which is a blessing (or a curse). That is, you will be given a general idea of what you should be eating and what you should avoid, but whether or not you follow it, and to what degree you do, is entirely up to you. Those who like cooking may find this to be particularly appealing; after all, it implies that this diet allows you entire creative flexibility when it comes to the foods you prepare and consume. The fact that there is no specific meal plan to follow or calorie count to adhere to can be disheartening if you are just starting started, or if you aren't especially fond of cooking.

The fact is that this is really a positive development since it implies that you will never get bored with your meals! They're also fairly filling, so you can eat as much as you want of them (without going overboard). You could probably eat something new every day for a couple of years and still not run out of recipes, but that is entirely up to you and your preferences! For those who want a more structured meal plan, you may just design your own. Consider creating a menu that will last for two to three weeks, and then repeating it until you feel the need to switch things up - but you will have to come up with the ideas for these dishes on your own.

The following are the foods that you should consume when on a weight loss program:

Meat, poultry, and seafood are examples of what is considered "fresh."

Whole grains are a kind of grain that has all of the nutrients found in grains.

Legumes

fruit that has been picked recently

Vegetables that are in season.

Nuts and seeds are good sources of protein.

Fats that are good for you.

Take advantage of your next shopping trip to stock up on all of these healthy whole foods. You have complete control over how elaborate or simple your meals are since the components are quite basic. There are no longer any justifications. Depending on where you live, certain items may not be as readily accessible as others, or they may be more costly, but the goal is to make do with what you have on hand. To be sure, it's preferable if you can adhere to Mediterranean-style foods as much as possible; but, it's quite OK to stuff your face with locally sourced fruits and veggies rather than French fries. Local products and ingredients are acceptable as long as you adhere to the basic principles of the Mediterranean eating plan as closely as possible.

However, you should be cautious about taking advantage of the fact that the diet is not restricted. Aside from that, avoid getting around it every other day by faking your way through. The Mediterranean diet, although it may be tough at first, is just as successful as your willingness to stick to it over the long term. Because it is considered a lifelong diet rather than a monthly or weekly challenge, it is referred to as a lifestyle change. It's important to realize that, even if you aren't very enthused about beginning this diet, it will allow you to have more control over what and how much you consume. You won't go hungry, and you won't have to give up carbohydrates or protein. You also won't have to limit your diet to solely salads and juices, as some people believe. Dietary flexibility is a strong point of this plan.

Things to strive to restrict as much as possible, and fully avoid if at all feasible, include the following.

meats of the red kind

Produce derived from poultry or dairy

Grains that have been processed

Sugar that has been refined

Fats that are not good for you

If you're having trouble coming up with ideas, here's a list to help you out.

beef, veal, and pig are the most common meats consumed in the US.

Chicken and turkey are both good options.

Cheese, butter, cream, and milk are some of the most popular dairy products in America.

Blanching the grains of wheat (white flour, blanching the grains of rice)

Baking goods such as cookies and cakes, pastries, candy bars, soda and juice are also available.

Deep-fried doughnuts and donut holes, ice cream, and potato chips are some of the treats available.

Greek yogurt and eggs, on the other hand, are exempt from the ban. Including them in your diet shouldn't pose any problems as long as they are done moderately. Similarly, if you do decide to consume any of these items, do so in moderation and no more than a couple of times each month. It is recommended that you consume chicken or turkey instead of beef or pig when it comes to animal protein. The Mediterranean Diet's foundational ingredients

Chapter 2

Despite the fact

Despite the fact that we have discussed the types of meals you should consume while on the diet, it is now time to dig into the nitty-gritty and give a face to the titles of the ingredients. As previously said, the Mediterranean diet emphasizes the consumption of whole foods that are easy to prepare and prepare. Even if Ancient Greece had speciality stores where you could purchase hundreds of imported substitutes for the same product, we find it hard to believe. Additionally, the upper class was quite tiny in comparison to the rest of the population, indicating that the Mediterranean diet was more of a middle-class eating pattern than an entirely higher-class eating pattern, as previously stated.

Having said that, for the most part, we'll be sticking to basic essentials. In any case, this does not rule out more complicated meals or the opportunity to experiment with other components if that is what you are interested in. Our point is simply that the Mediterranean diet is fundamentally easy, and you don't need to make it any more complicated than you really do unless you really want to.

Generally speaking, we will be using foods that are indigenous to the Mediterranean region. Please keep in mind that the meals you will be cooking are typically low in sodium as well, but they will be just as tasty since they place a strong emphasis on the use of spices and herbs to flavor their dishes. It is amazing what a little garlic, parsley, basil, and paprika can do, even if you are not a big fan of the kitchen. The main food categories you should be eating, on the other hand, are whole worlds in their own right, and we are going to help you break down precisely what each of them should consist of in order to make your gastronomic journey a lot easier and your excursions to the store a lot shorter.

As an example, consider the following types of fish and seafood.

The salmon and tuna are the most popular fish in the Pacific (fresh, not canned)

Mackerel\sSardines

Tilapia, eel, and sea bass are some of the most popular seafood choices.

Shrimp\sSquid

Octopus\sOysters\sMussels

Crab\sClam

Despite the fact that fresh fish is always preferred, we will not be fussy if the only seafood available is frozen. Make certain, however, that it is not breaded, seasoned, or otherwise processed in any manner before consuming it! Be as natural as possible with your expression!

Whole grains include, for example:

Oatmeal

Brown rice is a kind of rice that has a nutty flavor and is low in carbohydrates.

Pappardelle with whole grain

Millet

Couscous

Bulger

Barley

Bread made with whole grains

Barley\sBuckwheat Fats that are considered to be beneficial include:

Olive oil is a kind of oil that comes from the olive fruit.

Omega-3 fatty acids are found in flaxseed oil, which is also known as flaxseed oil

Biodiesel made from soya beans. Nuts and seeds include the following:

Almonds

Walnuts

Hazelnuts

Macadamias

Peanuts

Cashews

Nosegay nuts are a kind of pine nuts that are native to Southeast Asia.

Pistachios

Safflower seeds are one of the most common types of seeds found in the sunflower family.

seeds of chia

Flaxseed

Make sure to get unsalted nuts and seeds while you are out shopping.

Fruits that are examples:

Dates

Figs\sApricots

Apples

Grapes

Melon

Pomegranate

Peaches

Clementine Vegetable examples include:

Tomatoes

Zucchinis

Mushrooms (Portobello)

Eggplant

Carrots

Red onions are a kind of onion that grows in a bunch of different colors and shapes.

Peppers (bell) Legumes include, for example, the following.

Cannellini beans are a kind of bean that is native to Italy and are used for a variety of purposes.

Chickpeas

Lentils

Beans that have been soaked in a nitrate solution

Especially when it comes to canned legumes, there are many different alternatives available on the market. We're not going to say no to canned beans outright, but we do recommend that you use them in moderation or for last-minute meals when you're too exhausted to prepare. The key is to thoroughly rinse and drain them so that you can completely remove all of the sodium and salt from the solution they were in before you cook them. Nonetheless, we will state that it is always preferable to get raw versions if available, and just soak them overnight in warm water before cooking. Besides being healthier and yielding more servings, it is also substantially less expensive than purchasing canned beans on a consistent basis.

Herbs and spices include the following:

Parsley\sMint

Basil

Thyme

Paprika

Garlic

Cumin

Fennel

Dill

Rosemary

Fresh garlic is always the best, but when it comes to other herbs and spices, we won't be as fussy as we are with the fresh garlic. Purchase them whole or ground, depending on which you would use the most. Spices that have been ground are preferable, according to our opinion. Despite the fact that they lose their flavor after a while, we find them to be far more convenient than fresh herbs and spices, which tend to go bad very quickly. In this case, dried and ground herbs and spices may be your best option unless you're making your own basil pesto. Dishes for Sauces, Dipping Sauces, and Dressings, Chapter 1 Cooking Time: 10 minutes for the Chimichurri Sauce 8 portions (per serving)

Ingredients:

olive oil (approximately a 12-cup quantity)

vinegar made from grapes, 1/3 cup red wine minced 4 garlic cloves (peeled and peeled),

12 cup finely chopped fresh parsley (optional).

12 cup finely chopped fresh coriander 1 tablespoon oregano leaves (freshly chopped)

Red pepper flakes (about 12 teaspoon) depending on the situation

Blend all of the ingredients in a blender until they are completely smooth.

Now that the sauce has been prepared, you can use it!
Per serving, the following nutritional information: Nutritional Values: 116 Calories

12.7 g of fat (net) 0.8 g of carbohydrate 1.3 g of carbohydrate

0.5 g of fiber

0.1 gram of sugar

0.3 g of protein

23.5 milligrams sodium

Cooking Time: 10 minutes for the Avgolemono Sauce The following ingredients are used in the preparation of four servings:

Separate 2 or 3 large eggs, separating the yolks from the whites Chicken broth (114-112 cups)

Fresh lemon juice (4-6 tablespoons) 1/4 cup (of liquid)

Directions:

The egg whites should be placed in a clean glass bowl and whisked until foamy.

Mix together the egg yolks, broth, lemon juice and water in a separate mixing bowl until everything is thoroughly mixed.

Gently fold in the whipped egg whites until they are fully incorporated into the batter.

Now that the sauce has been prepared, you can use it! Per serving, the following nutritional information: 53% of your daily caloric intake

3.1 g of fat (total) 0.9 g of carbohydrate 1.25 g of carbohydrate

0.1 g of fiber

0.9% of your daily caloric intake

4.9 g of protein

278 milligrams of sodium

Cooking Time: 10 minutes for the Zhug Sauce 8 portions (per serving)

Ingredients:

6-inch long piece of jalapeo pepper, sliced peeled and minced two garlic cloves cup fresh cilantro leaves (to taste) teaspoon salt

parsley leaves (about 12 cup)

12 teaspoon coriander leaves, finely chopped

Cumin (ground) – 12 teaspoon

green cardamom, ground to a fine powder, 12 teaspoon Extra-virgin olive oil (about 1/3 cup) fresh lemon juice (about 2 tablespoons)

Directions:

Chop the jalapenos, garlic, and salt until coarsely chopped in a food processor until everything is well combined.

Process until a thick paste forms, adding in the fresh herbs and spices as needed.

Into a mixing bowl, add the herb paste.

In a medium-sized mixing bowl, combine the oil and lemon juice until fully combined.

Now that the sauce has been prepared, you can use it! Per serving, the following nutritional information: calories: 82 fat grams: 8.7 net calories: 82 0.9 g of carbohydrate Sugars: 1.6 g carbohydrate

0.7 g of fiber

1 g Sugars 1 g Carbohydrates 0.4 g Protein

299 milligrams of sodium

Ten minutes are required to prepare the tartamasalata sauce. The following ingredients are used in this recipe:

approximately 12 cup water, 1/12 of a red onion, chopped

a quarter cup of olive oil 4 white sandwich bread slices

tarama (white): 3 tablespoons (fish roe) lemon juice (about 2 tbsp. fresh) cup sunflower oil and a pinch of sugar

Directions:

Blend the onion and water together until smooth in a blender.

Pour the onion puree into a mixing bowl using a strainer.

Using a food processor, puree the onion and add the bread slices, olive oil, tarama, lemon juice, sugar, and salt until smooth.

Continue to run the motor while adding the sunflower oil in small amounts at a time, pulsing until fully combined.

Now that the sauce has been prepared, you can use it! Per serving, the following nutritional information: Energy intake: 170 calories

The following is the net amount of fat: 17.2 g 3.7 g of carbohydrate 3.8 g of carbohydrate

0.1 g of fiber

0.5 g of sucrose

1.1 g of protein

42 mg of sodium

Amba Sauce is a type of sauce that is made from a variety of herbs and vegetables.

15 minutes are required for preparation. Approximately 6 minutes of preparation time 16 portions (per serving)

Mangoes, peeled and pitted, and cut into chunks are the primary ingredients. depending on the situation

grapeseed oil (1/4 cup)

the hot paprika, 2 tablespoons 2 teaspoons cumin seed (or equivalent)

tablespoon ground turmeric 1 teaspoon mustard seed 1 teaspoon cumin Fenugreek seeds (ground) 1 teaspoon

12 teaspoon coriander leaves, finely chopped

12 tsp. ground black pepper, if desired brown sugar, 6-8 garlic cloves (minced), 6 tablespoons

11-cup water is an appropriate amount.

Directions:

Gently toss the mango pieces and salt together in a large mixing bowl until everything is evenly coated with dressing.

In a jar, combine the mango pieces and set it out in the sun for approximately 5 days.

In a separate bowl, drain the mango pieces and set aside the juice.

Using parchment paper, arrange the mango pieces and set them aside for approximately 3-4 hours.

In a small skillet, heat the oil over medium heat and cook the spices for about 1-2 minutes, stirring frequently.

Cook for about 2-3 minutes, stirring constantly, until the garlic and brown sugar are fragrant.

In a medium-sized mixing bowl, combine the mango pieces, reserved juices, and water until everything is well combined.

With an immersion blender, smooth out the sauce once it has been removed from the heat source.

To serve, transfer the sauce to a serving bowl and set it aside to cool completely before using.

Per serving, the following nutritional information:

Nutritional Values: 68 calories

3.9 g of fat (net). 7.7 g of carbohydrate 8.9 g of carbohydrate

1.2 g of fiber

7 g of sucrose

0.7 g of protein

14.4 milligrams (mg) sodium

Cooking Time: 15 minutes for the Romesco Sauce 10 portions (per person).

Ingredients:

14.4 ounces can of fire-roasted tomatoes, drained 12.4 ounce can of diced roasted red peppers (drained) 1-2 garlic cloves, minced 34.4 cup raw blanched almonds, toasted 14.4 cup raw blanched hazelnuts, toasted 14.4 cup fresh parsley, minced 14.4 cup extra-virgin olive oil

lemon juice (about 1 tablespoon) tablespoon balsamic vinegar 1 teaspoon paprika smoked 1 teaspoon red wine vinegar

Crushed red pepper flakes (112 to 1 tablespoon) depending on the situation

Directions:

Blend the ingredients in a food processor until they are completely smooth.

Now that the sauce has been prepared, you can use it! Per serving, the following nutritional information: Calories in a serving (148 calories)

Nutritional Information: 9.9 g fat, 8.2 g net carbs 9.9 g of carbohydrate

1.5 g of sugar and 1.7 grams of fiber.

35 grams of protein

359 milligrams of sodium

Cooking Time: 15 minutes for the Tomato Sauce Approximately 13 minutes for preparation. Ingredients: 112 tablespoons extra-virgin olive oil (servings: four) plum tomatoes, seeded and finely chopped, 112 teaspoons butter cups 1 onion, peeled and minced 3 garlic cloves

1 12 tablespoon capers 1 tablespoon Dijon mustard

fresh parsley (11 1/2 tablespoons chopped) 14 teaspoon crushed red pepper flakes 112 tablespoons fresh chives (minced) Season with salt and freshly ground black pepper to taste.

Directions:

Stir frequently while cooking the tomatoes for about 6 minutes in a medium wok over medium-high heat, infusing the olive oil with butter.

Bring the stock to a boil while stirring in the garlic, capers, and mustard.

Stir occasionally while cooking for about 2 minutes on low heat or until the sauce has slightly thickened.

Remove the pan from the heat and add the remaining ingredients, stirring until well combined..

Before serving, allow the dish to cool.

Chapter 3

Breakfast Recipes

Preparation Time: 10 minutes for Apricot Walnut Yogurt Bowl Recipe serves 2 people; ingredients are as follows.

Greek yogurt (plain) - 1 cup

3 cups dried apricots, diced roughly 2 cups toasted walnuts, diced 2 tablespoons honey

Method: Divide the yogurt and apricots among serving bowls and stir until everything is evenly distributed.

Honey should be drizzled over the top and walnuts should be sprinkled on.

Serve as soon as possible after preparing it. Per serving, the following nutritional information: 207 Calories per serving

6.8 g (net) of total fat 26.1 g of carbohydrate 26.7 g of carbohydrate

2.6 g of fiber

23.9 g of sucrose

10.2 g of protein

Amount of sodium in one serving is 88 mg.

Cherry Pomegranate is a fruit that is derived from the fruit cherry. Approximately 10 minutes are required for preparation of the smoothie bowl. 4 individual servings

Ingredients:

Blend all of the ingredients together in a blender until they are smooth and creamy.

Frozen dark sweet cherries (16 ounces) 1 (16-ounce bag) Plain Greek yogurt (11 1/2 cups)

the juice from one quarter cup of pomegranates Milk, one-third cup

vanilla extract (about 1 teaspoon)

ground cinnamon (about 34 teaspoon) the equivalent of six ice cubes

As a finishing touch, we've included some suggestions.

12 cup pomegranate seeds (freshly harvested)

Pistachios (about 12 cup), finely chopped

Directions:

The ingredients for the smoothie bowl should be placed in a high-speed blender and blended until smooth.

Using a slotted spoon, distribute the mixture among the four serving bowls.

Serve the pomegranate seeds and pistachios on top of each bowl as soon as they are prepared.

Per serving, the following nutritional information:

The calories in this recipe are 261 calories.

5.2 g of fat (net). 42.7 g of carbohydrates 46.22 g of carbohydrate

3.5 g of fiber

398.8 g of sucrose

8.9 g of protein

Amount of sodium in one serving: 118 mg

Preparation Time for Raspberry Muesli: 5 minutes

Ingredients: 34 cup muesli, 2 servings

freshly picked raspberries (about 1 cup total) 12-cups low-fat milk is a serving size.

Method: Divide the muesli among serving bowls and garnish with raspberries.

After that, pour in the milk and put the bowl down.

Per serving, the following nutritional information: Nutritional Values: 224 calories

4.2 g of fat (total) 33,5 g of carbohydrate 40.55 g of carbohydrate

7.8 g of fibre

18.2 g of sucrose

9.9 g of protein

Sodium intake: 151 milligrams

Porridge with Quinoa and Apples

Approximately 10 minutes are required for preparation.

Approximately 1 minute of preparation time 6 portions (per serving)

Ingredients:

water (114 cup)

apple juice (around 1 cup)

uncooked quinoa (rinsed): 12 cups Honey and cinnamon stick (about a tablespoon each) apples, cored and diced with a pinch of salt

Method: Place all of the ingredients (save the apples) in the Instant Pot and stir to incorporate well.

Close the lid and adjust the vent to a position that is completely sealed.

1 minute at high pressure using the "Manual" setting on the stovetop

Then, after the cooking time is up, hit "Cancel" and gently push the button labeled "Quick."

Fork fluff the quinoa after the cover has been removed.

Immediately transfer the porridge to serving dishes and top with apple slices to serve right away.

Per serving, the following nutritional information:

calories: 225 fat grams: 2.8 grams net carbohydrate grams: 40.2 cals Sugars: 14.6 g Carbohydrates (45.1) Fiber (4.9) Protein (6.2) Calories (6.4)

Sodium intake: 132 milligrams

Porridge with Barley

Approximately 10 minutes are required for preparation. Approximately 20 minutes for preparation. The following ingredients are used in the preparation of four servings:

Pearl Barley (about 1 cup). 3-gallon bucket (of milk)

14.4 cups dried dates (pitted and diced) 14.4 cups agave nectar bananas, peeled and cut into two tiny pieces

1 cup walnuts (chopped), 4 teaspoons

In an instant pot, add all of the ingredients (except the walnuts) and cook on high for 2 minutes, or on low for 3 minutes.

Close the lid and adjust the vent to a position that is completely sealed.

Cook for 20 minutes at "High Pressure" on "Manual" setting on your stove.

After the cooking time has expired, press "Cancel" and then "Natural" to release the pressure in the pressure cooker.

Take off the cover and thoroughly stir the barley mixture with a spoon.

Transfer the porridge to serving dishes and top with banana slices and walnuts to serve immediately, if possible.

Per serving, the following nutritional information:

The calories in this recipe are 452 calories.

9.1 g of fat per serving Nutrients: zero grams of carbohydrate 84.5 g of carbohydrates

11.5 g of fiber

37 g of sugar

13.7 g of protein

Amount of sodium in one serving: 92 mg

a porridge made with dried fruits

15 minutes are required for preparation. Approximately 20 minutes for preparation. Recipe serves 6 people; ingredients are as follows.

1 cup rolled oats (old-fashioned)

12 cup rinsed quinoa (optional)

12 cup rolled wheat flakes 14 cup chia seeds 14 cup chopped dried apricots Dried cranberries, 2 teaspoons raisins (about 2 tablespoons)

12-teaspoon cinnamon powder

sodium bicarbonate (salt): 12 teaspoon Milk, 712 to 8 cups

Maple syrup (4-6 tablespoons) 2 cups of fresh berries in various combinations

1 cup walnuts (chopped), 6 teaspoons

Instructions: In a medium-sized saucepan, combine the oats, quinoa, wheat flakes, chia seeds, dried fruit, cinnamon, salt, and milk and bring to a boil over medium-high heat.

Stir regularly while cooking over low heat for approximately 12-15 minutes or until the sauce has thickened, partly covered.

Set aside, covered, for about 5 minutes after removing from the heat.

Remove the lid and mix in the maple syrup until well incorporated.

Serve with a berry and walnut streusel on top to complete the presentation.

Per serving, the following nutritional information:

There are 421 calories in this recipe.

15 g fat, 51.2 g carbohydrate net (total). 58.6 g of carbohydrates

7.4 g of fiber

27.7 g of sucrose

18.1 g of protein

Three hundred and forty-one milligrams of sodium

Tomatoes and eggs are a traditional combination.

Approximately 15 minutes are required for preparation.

Approximately 16 minutes for preparation. 4 individual servings

Ingredients:

1 cup extra-virgin olive oil 2 tablespoons adobo

1/2 a green bell pepper, seeded and finely diced 1 medium yellow onion, peeled and finely minced

depending on the situation 2 romain lettuce leaves

1 cup tomato paste (optional)

12 teaspoon oregano leaves (dry), chopped aleppo pepper (about 1 tablespoon)

black peppercorns (to taste) if necessary Beat four big eggs until they are light and fluffy.

Cook the bell pepper, onion, and salt for approximately 4-5 minutes in a 10-inch wok over medium heat until the vegetables are soft.

Cook for approximately 5-7 minutes, stirring regularly, after which add the tomatoes, tomato paste, oregano, Aleppo pepper, and black pepper.

With the help of a spoon, push the tomato mixture to one side of the pan and immediately reduce the heat to medium.

Cook for about 2-3 minutes, stirring gently and consistently, until the egg is set in the middle.

Cook for approximately 1 minute, stirring constantly, until the tomato mixture is fully cooked.

Hot food should be served.

Per serving, the following nutritional information:

Nutritional Values: 174 calories

12 g fat, 7.7 g carbohydrate (net carbohydrate) 10.1 g of carbohydrate

Amounts of fiber and sugar are as follows: (2.4 g)

8 grams of protein

Sodium intake: 126 milligrams

Approximately 15 minutes to prepare the chicken and bell pepper omelet. 23 and a half hours of preparation time 1 cup each person; 5 cups total.

Ingredients:

Cooking spray that is non-stick

Milk (one-and-a-half cups) There are 6 eggs in this recipe.

134 teaspoon red pepper flakes, crushed 14 teaspoon red pepper flakes, crushed 1 garlic clove, minced 12 teaspoon dry parsley Season with salt and freshly ground black pepper to taste.

one large red bell pepper, seeded and thinly sliced one cup cooked chicken, chopped small white onion, finely chopped 1 medium white onion, finely chopped

a cup of shredded mozzarella cheese

Directions:

Cooking spray should be used to lightly coat the bottom of the slow cooker.

Using a mixer on low speed, whip the milk until it is completely incorporated with the eggs, garlic, parsley, red pepper flakes, salt, and black pepper.

The egg mixture should be placed in the slow cooker that has been preheated and is ready.

Stir in the chicken, bell pepper, and onion until everything is well-combined and heated through.

Slow-cook for 2 12 hours on "High" setting in a covered slow cooker.

Uncover the slow cooker after the cooking time has been finished and evenly sprinkle the omelet with cheese.

Continue to simmer for 15 minutes on "High" in the slow cooker with the lid ajar once more.

Uncover the slow cooker after the cooking time has been finished and transfer the omelet to a serving platter.

Make wedges of similar size and serve immediately.

Per serving, the following nutritional information:

Nutritional information per serving: 150 calories

7.5 g of fat per serving Nutrients: zero grams of carbohydrate 5.2 g of carbohydrate

0.7 g of fiber

3.3 g of sucrose

15.6 g of protein

165 mg of sodium

Recipes for Meze, Tapas, and Antipasti are included in Chapter 3 of this cookbook.

Time Required for Preparation: 15 minutes for a Fruit, Nut, and Pickles Platter 10 portions (per person).

Ingredients:

Extra-virgin olive oil (around 12 cups)

12 cup mustard (Dijon)

fresh rosemary, minced (about 2-3 teaspoons) Season with salt and freshly ground black pepper to taste. one 10-ounce package of breadsticks (about

olives (about 1 cup) kalamata

12 cup pickled dill

Drained marinated artichoke hearts from a 6-ounce jar Pickled veggies, 1 (12-ounce) jar

Sun-dried tomatoes packed in olive oil, drained to 12 cup total 1 pear, peeled and cored; 1 apple, peeled and cored;

12 cup pitted dates 14 cup almonds 12 cup dates, pitted cashews (14 cup)

Cups of feta cheese (crumbled) 14 cup hazelnuts 14 cup pine nuts

Method: In a mixing bowl, combine the oil, the dijon and the rosemary along with the salt, black pepper, and a pinch of salt. Stir well to blend.

Place the rest of the ingredients on a serving plate and serve immediately thereafter.

Toss with the mustard sauce and serve immediately thereafter.

Calories and Nutritional Values per Serving

There are 391 calories in this recipe.

26.3% of total calories come from fat. Sugars: 28.2 g Carbohydrates 33.4 g of carbohydrates

5.2 g of fiber

13.3 g of sugar

9.9 g of protein

1003 milligrams of sodium

In 15 minutes, you can have your chicken wings platter ready. Approximately 50 minutes for preparation. 6 portions (per serving)

Ingredients:

In the case of chicken wings, use the following ingredients.

Extra-virgin olive oil (around 12 cups)

fresh lemon juice (about 12 cups)

Peeled and smashed garlic cloves (six), Grated lemon zest (about 3 to 4 tablespoons) oregano leaves (112 tablespoon)

1 teaspoon paprika rojo (sweet)

Season with salt and freshly ground black pepper to taste.
3-pound boneless skinless chicken wings

16 ounces plain Greek yogurt (for the yogurt sauce).

lemon juice (about 2 tbsp. fresh) the finely minced garlic from 2 garlic cloves

depending on the situation

Regarding the preparation of the meal

12 cup of crumbled feta cheese

3-4 tablespoons finely chopped fresh parsley 2 lemons, cut 3-4 tablespoons fresh parsley

Directions:

Add all of the ingredients except the wings to a large mixing bowl and thoroughly combine.

In a large mixing bowl, combine all of the ingredients.

Let marinate overnight in the refrigerator.

400 degrees Fahrenheit is the recommended temperature for the oven.

Using a wide baking sheet, spread out the chicken wings so that they are all in one layer.

Preparation time: 45-50 minutes at 350 degrees F.

The wings should be placed aside for about 5 minutes after they have been removed from the oven.

The yogurt sauce may be made in the meanwhile by mixing together all of the ingredients in a large mixing basin.

Toss the wings with the feta and parsley before serving them on a plate.

Serve with a dollop of yogurt sauce and a few lemon wedges on the side for garnish.

Calories and Nutritional Values per Serving

Approximately 677 calories.

376 g (net) of fat 7.5 g of carbohydrate 8.5 g of carbohydrate

0.9 g of fiber

6.5% of the total calories are from sugar.

72.3 g of protein

163 milligrams of sodium

Chapter 4

Smoked Salmon Platter

Preparation time for the Smoked Salmon Platter: 15 minutes
Recipe serves 6 people; ingredients are as follows.

  Cream cheese, softened 4 ounces 1 tablespoon crushed red
pepper flakes (optional) depending on the situation
  smoked salmon (around 12 ounces) four eggs, peeled and
cut into slices, three cups feta cheese, cubed 1 finely sliced
cucumber (optional)
  1 bell pepper, seeded and finely sliced (about 1 cup) 1
medium-sized tomato, thinly sliced
  5 finely sliced radishes (optional)
  artichoke hearts marinated in a third cup of oil
  14 cup a variety of olives
  1 small red onion, thinly sliced 1 small yellow onion, thinly
sliced 1 lemon, peeled and cut into wedges
  To make the cream cheese, combine the cream cheese, red
pepper flakes, and salt in a small bowl and whisk until smooth.

Place the rest of the ingredients on a serving plate and serve immediately thereafter.

Serve with the cream cheese mixture on the side.

Calories and Nutritional Values per Serving

Calories in a serving: 245

15.8 g of fat (net) carbohydrate gramage: 6 gramage 8 grams of carbohydrates

2 g of dietary fiber

2.7 g of sugar

18.6 grams of protein

Sodium: 1033 milligrams

Platter with Tuna and Potatoes from Chapter 5: Poultry Recipes

Preparation time for the herb-crusted whole chicken: 15 minutes Approximately 50 minutes for preparation. 6 portions (per serving)

Ingredients:

Remove the neck and giblets from a whole chicken (four pounds). 1 (1-inch-long) piece of fresh ginger, chopped

4 garlic cloves, peeled and chopped

1 tiny bunch of fresh thyme (about)

1 tiny bunch of fresh rosemary (about)

a quarter teaspoon of paprika

Cumin (ground) – 12 teaspoon

Season with salt and freshly ground black pepper to taste.

14 cup freshly squeezed lemon juice 3 tablespoons extra-virgin olive oil

Directions: Place the chicken breast-side down on a large chopping board and set aside.

Start at the thigh and cut down one side of the backbone, then flip the bird around with a kitchen shear to finish the job.

Now, cut down the opposite side of the backbone and discard it.

Change the side and open it up like a book for a different look.

To flatten the backbone, pound it with force.

In a food processor, combine all of the ingredients (apart from the chicken) and process until completely smooth.

Add the marinade mixture to a large baking dish and set aside.

Add the chicken and liberally cover it with the marinade.

Cover the baking dish with plastic wrap and place it in the refrigerator overnight to marinate.

Preheat your oven to 450 degrees Fahrenheit.

In a roasting pan, arrange a rack of ribs.

Remove the chicken from the refrigerator and discard any extra marinade. Set the chicken aside to cool.

Place the chicken on a rack over a roasting pan, skin side down, and cook for 30 minutes.

25 minutes in the oven should enough.

Roast for another 25 minutes after flipping the chicken.

The chicken should be placed on a tray for approximately 10 minutes before carving after it has been removed from the oven.

Cut the chicken into desired-sized pieces with a knife and place them on a serving platter.

Per serving, the following nutritional information:

Calories in a serving: 644

Fat: 29.6 g net (total) Sugars: 1 gram Carbohydrates Sugars: 1.6 g carbohydrate

0.5 g of fiber

0.3 g of sugar

Protein content: 87.8 g

Sodium: 290 milligrams

Whole Chicken with Tomato Stuffing

Time required for preparation: 20 minutes Preparation time: 2 hours 6 portions (per serving)

Ingredients:

1 cup crumbled feta cheese (optional) pine nuts (about a third of a cup)

a third cup of chopped and drained tomatoes

14 cup sun-dried tomatoes in olive oil, finely diced 6 garlic cloves, peeled and minced

1 tablespoon dried oregano leaves, finely chopped extra-virgin olive oil (about a third cup)

red pepper flakes, roughly chopped (about 1 tablespoon) Season with salt and freshly ground black pepper to taste.

Remove the neck and giblets from a 4 pound whole chicken.
1 lemon, peeled and sliced in half

1 cup Marsala wine (optional)

6 Yukon gold potatoes (yukon gold potatoes are a kind of potato that is native to Canada).

Directions:

Preheat the oven to 425 degrees Fahrenheit.

In a large mixing bowl, combine the feta, pine nuts, chopped tomatoes, sun-dried tomatoes, garlic, 1 tablespoon oregano, and 1 tablespoon olive oil, stirring well to combine the ingredients.

To make the sauce, combine 2 tablespoons oil, red pepper flakes, salt, and black pepper in a small dish.

Rub the chicken with the cut edges of the lemon halves and then with the olive oil mixture, rubbing it in well.

Fill the cavity of the bird with the tomato mixture and bake for 30 minutes.

Make a securing seal around the cavity of the chicken with a few toothpicks.

Place the chicken breast side down in a roasting pan and cook for 30 minutes.

40 minutes in the oven should enough.

The chicken should be placed breast side up in the roasting pan once it has been removed from the oven.

Pour the wine over the chicken and let it sit for a few minutes.

Cook for 20 minutes at 350°F.

Meanwhile, combine the potatoes, remaining oil, salt, and black pepper in a large mixing basin and well combine.

The potatoes should be placed in the bottom of a big baking dish.

Take the chicken roasting pan out of the oven and set it aside.

Half of the liquid should be removed from the roasting pan and poured over the potatoes.

Place the chicken on top of the potatoes, breast side up, and serve immediately.

Pour the remainder of the liquid from the roasting pan over the chicken and bake for another 30 minutes.

30 minutes in the oven should enough.

Remove the baking dish from the oven and place the chicken on a serving tray to cool slightly.

Wrap the chicken in aluminum foil to keep it from drying out.

Transfer the baking dish to the oven once again and roast the potatoes for another 30 minutes or until they are tender.

Using scissors, cut the chicken into desired-sized pieces and arrange them beside the potatoes.

Per serving, the following nutritional information:

Calories in a serving: 953

60 g of fat (net) g of carbohydrates (32.1 g) 57.7 g carbohydrate calories

3.6 g of dietary fiber

3.6 g of sugar

62.16 g of protein

Sodium: 570 milligrams

Recipes for Red Meat (Chapter 6)

Leg of Lamb Braised in Red Wine

15 minutes are required for preparation. Preparation time: 4 hours and 8 minutes

Ingredients: 8 servings (serves 8)

1 (3-pound) boneless leg of lamb, cut to desired thickness Season with salt and freshly ground black pepper to taste.

5 tbsp. extra-virgin olive oil (distributed evenly). 6 finely sliced garlic cloves (around 6 cloves total)

lemon juice (about 2 tbsp. fresh) 6 garlic cloves, peeled and minced

2 teaspoons thyme leaves (fresh)

dried rosemary (about 2 teaspoons) 1 teaspoon oregano leaves (dried)

Sweet paprika, 1/4 teaspoon (or as desired)

peeling and dicing one pound pearl onions red wine (dry) 1 cup

beef broth (around 12 cup)

Directions:

Use a lot of salt and black pepper while seasoning the leg of lamb!

For up to 1 hour, leave the dish at room temperature.

A big wok or skillet heated to medium heat should be used to sear the lamb for around 7-8 minutes, or until it is thoroughly browned.

Set aside to cool gently after removing from the heat.

Cut incisions into the lamb on both sides with a sharp knife. Set aside.

In each slit, place a sliver of garlic to flavor the space.

In a small mixing bowl, combine the remaining oil, lemon juice, minced garlic, herbs, and paprika, stirring well to combine all the ingredients.

Spread the oil mixture evenly over the leg of lamb.

Place the pearl onions, wine, and broth in a slow cooker and set it on low for 8 hours or overnight.

Place the leg of lamb on top of the gratin and serve immediately.

Slow-cook for about 3-4 hours on "High" setting in a covered slow-cooker.

Then, using two tongs, carefully move the leg of lamb to a serving tray when the cooking time has been finished in the slow cooker.

Serve immediately with pan juices on the side of the plate.

Calories and Nutritional Values per Serving

Calories: 450

net amount of fat: 21.4 g 5.9 g of carbohydrate 7.6 g of carbohydrate

The following nutrients are included: fiber (1.7 grams), sugar (2.8 grams), and protein (48.8 grams).

194 milligrams of sodium

Lamb Shanks with Artichokes is a delicious dish to make for any occasion.

15 minutes are required for preparation. 1414 hours of cooking time 6 portions (per serving)

Ingredients:

lamb shanks, cooked in a French style

teaspoons olive oil (divided) 14 cup flour 1 large can marinated artichoke hearts (14-ounce) 2 onions, cut garlic cloves, finely sliced (14-ounce)

teaspoons grated lemon rind (optional) 34 cup pitted Kalamata olives

Fresh oregano (chopped): 1 tbsp

Season with salt and freshly ground black pepper to taste.

White wine (about 12 cup)

chicken broth (212 cups)

Directions:

Lamb shanks and flour should be placed in a big plastic bag.

Seal the bag and shake it to coat the contents with the coating solution.

Sautee the lamb shanks for approximately 4-5 minutes each batch in a big skillet with 2 teaspoons of oil, turning once, until they are browned on both sides.

Transfer the shanks onto a serving plate using a slotted spoon.

The onions and garlic should be sautéed for around 4-5 minutes in the same pan with the remaining oil on medium heat.

Immediately remove the pan from the stovetop or oven.

Place the lamb shanks and onion mixture in a slow cooker and set it on low for 8 hours.

Stir in the remaining ingredients once you've finished assembling the cake.

Preparing the dish in the slow cooker takes around 4 hours on "High."

Uncover the slow cooker after the cooking time is over and serve immediately.

Calories and Nutritional Values per Serving

Energy: 710 calories

20.4% of total calories come from fat. 12.8 g of carbohydrates 17.9 grams of carbohydrates

The following nutrients are included in this food: fiber (5.1 g) sugar (2.8 g)

85.1 g of protein, 772 mg of sodium

Pot Roast with Beans (Lamb Shank)

15 minutes are required for preparation. Approximately 1 hour and 5 minutes of preparation time

4 individual servings

Ingredients:

4 lamb shanks (each weighing 10 ounces).

Season with salt and freshly ground black pepper to taste. 1 cup extra-virgin olive oil 2 tablespoons adobo

white wine (dry) 12 cup

half a medium-sized onion, cut into quarters the finely minced garlic from 2 garlic cloves

peeled and sliced into quarters 1 big carrot

quartered and fronds off 1 tiny fennel bulb reserved 2 sprigs of parsley

chicken broth (214 cups)

8 ounces dry cannellini beans, soaked in water for 24 hours, drained, and washed thereafter peeled and sliced one big carrot the equivalent of about 1 medium tomato, seeded, and chopped

Directions:

Season the lamb shanks with salt and freshly ground black pepper to your liking.

Cook for 2 hours at room temperature after covering the shanks with a piece of aluminum foil.

Press "Sauté" on the instant pot after adding in the oil. Then, in two batches, add the lamb shanks and fry for 3-4 minutes each side, depending on how thick they are.

Transfer the shanks to a serving platter using a slotted spoon to prevent sticking.

Scrape up any browned pieces from the bottom of the pot while you simmer the wine for approximately 3-4 minutes in a large saucepan.

Toss in the shanks, onion, quartered carrot, fennel, garlic, and bay leaf after pressing "Cancel."

Close the lid and adjust the vent to a position that is completely sealed.

"Manual" is selected, and the cooking time is 35 minutes at "High Pressure."

After the cooking time has expired, select "Cancel" and let the pressure to naturally relax for about 10 minutes before continuing. After then, do a "Quick" release of pressure.

Toss the shanks onto a platter with a slotted spoon when you've opened the cover.

Remove the veggies from the pan and return the liquid to the pan.

Stir in the beans, carrots, and tomato until everything is well-combined (about 5 minutes).

Close the lid and adjust the vent to a position that is completely sealed.

Bake at high pressure for 10 minutes on manual setting (or 10 minutes on high pressure on pressure cooker).

After the cooking time has expired, hit "Cancel" and perform a "Natural" release for the next 30 minutes.

It takes approximately ten minutes to complete the process. After then, do a "Quick" release of pressure.

Close and remove the lid from the pan, then transfer to serving bowls.

1 shank should be placed on top of each bowl before it is served.

Calories and Nutritional Values per Serving

A total of 733 calories are consumed.

net amount of fat: 29 g Sugars: 15.4 grams Carbohydrates 22.2 g of carbohydrate

6.8 g of fiber

5.4 g of sucrose

87 grams of protein

the following amounts of sodium: 889 mg

Cooking time for buttered lamb chops: 10 minutes. Approximately 13 minutes for preparation. 4 individual servings

Ingredients:

8 bone-in lamb loin chops (1 inch thick) with a sauce depending on the situation

black pepper (ground) 1 teaspoon olive oil (about 2 tbsp.

Salted butter, 4 tablespoons minced 4 garlic cloves (peeled and peeled),

chopped 1 tablespoon of fresh thyme

chopped fresh rosemary (about 1 tablespoon)

Directions:

Sea salt and black pepper should be sprinkled evenly over the lamb chops.

Cook the lamb chops for about 3-4 minutes per side in a large cast-iron wok over medium-high heat, turning halfway through.

Reduce the heat to medium-low after adding the butter, garlic, and fresh herbs.

Remove from heat and spoon butter sauce over chops every 5 minutes for approximately 5 minutes total time.

Hot food should be served.

Calories and Nutritional Values per Serving

Nutritional Values: 594 Calories

35.4 g of fat (total) carbohydrate grams: 1.5 grams carbohydrate grams: 2.3 grams carbohydrate grams: 1.5 grams carbohydrate grams

The following nutrients are included: fiber, sugar, and protein. Sodium is included in the following amounts: 294 mg.

Lamb Chops with Garlic and Chipotle Preparation Time: 10 minutes. Approximately 6 minutes of preparation time The following ingredients are used in the preparation of four servings:

Peeled and chopped garlic cloves depending on the situation

1/4 cup crushed, finely ground black mustard seeds ground cumin, 2 teaspoons

ground ginger (one teaspoon)

coriander leaves (ground) 1 teaspoon

12-teaspoon cinnamon powder black peppercorns (to taste) if necessary 8 lamb chops (4 ounces), trimmed and marinated

1 tablespoon extra-virgin olive oil 1 tablespoon lemon juice 1 tablespoon tarragon

Directions:

To prepare the garlic cloves, place them on a cutting board and sprinkle them with a little salt.

Squeeze the garlic until it forms a paste with the help of a knife.

Into a mixing bowl, add the garlic paste.

Mix in the spices and black pepper until everything is evenly distributed.

Slice both sides of the chops with a sharp knife, making 3-4 cuts each time.

Garlic mixture should be generously applied to the chops.

The chops should be cooked for approximately 3 minutes per side in a large cast-iron wok over medium heat.

Serve immediately after drizzling with lemon juice..

Nutritional Information per Serving Calories: 1 g Fat: 0 g Protein: 0 g Fat: 0 g Calories: 0 g 467

20.7% of calories come from fat, and 1.9 grams come from carbohydrate. 2.4 g of carbohydrate

The following nutrients are included: fiber (0.5 g), sugar (0.2 g), and vitamin C.

64.4 g of protein

214 milligrams of sodium

Prepare Lemony Lamb Chops in 10 Minutes Total Time: 10 Minutes Approximately 9 minutes for preparation. 4 individual servings

Ingredients:

Fresh lemon juice and 14 cup extra-virgin olive oil

chopped fresh oregano (about 2 tablespoons) 1 tablespoon minced garlic

Season with salt and freshly ground black pepper to taste. (4) lamb chops (each weighing 8 ounces and 12 inches thick).

Directions:

In a large mixing bowl, combine all of the ingredients except the chops and mix well.

To marinate the chops, place them in a large sealable plastic bag with the marinade.

Stir vigorously to coat everything evenly after sealing the bag.

Allow for about 1 hour of resting time at room temp.

The lamb chops should be removed from the bag and the marinade should be discarded.

To dry the lamb chops, pat them with paper towels.

With a pinch of salt, season the lamb chops.

2 lamb chops should be cooked for about 3 minutes on each side in a large cast-iron grill pan over medium-high heat, if possible.

Cook for approximately 3 more minutes after moving the lamb chops.

Adjust the heat to medium-low after flipping the lamb chops on their sides.

About 2-3 minutes should be sufficient.

Proceed to cook the remainder of the lamb chops in the same fashion.

Removing the lamb chops from the heat and allowing them to rest for approximately 5 minutes before serving

Calories and Nutritional Values per Serving

Nutritional Values: 540 calories

net amount of fat: 29.5 g 0.8 g of carbohydrate 1.8 g of carbohydrate

1 gram of fiber

The amount of sugar in this recipe is 0.3 g

64 grams of protein

213 milligrams of sodium

Rack of Lamb (also known as rack of lamb) is a type of lamb that is roasted on a rack and served with a side of mashed potatoes and vegetables.

15 minutes are required for preparation. Approximately 50 minutes for preparation. 6 portions (per serving)

Ingredients:

extra-virgin olive oil (approximately 12 cup plus 1 tablespoon) crushed garlic cloves (six total)

the leaves of 1 freshly chopped bunch of thyme

1. one bunch of freshly chopped rosemary

1/2 teaspoon red pepper flakes, crushed 2 (112-pound) lamb racks, frenched

Season with salt and freshly ground black pepper to taste.

Directions:

Mix together 12 cup of oil, the garlic, the fresh herbs, and the red pepper flakes in a large baking dish until everything is evenly distributed.

Make a well in the center of the marinade and pour in enough to cover the lamb racks.

Allow at least 6 hours of refrigeration time, flipping once or twice during that time.

Refrigerate for 1 hour before baking on a baking sheet that has been left out at room temperature for that time.

Preheat the oven to 275 degrees Fahrenheit (180 degrees Celsius).

Remove the lamb racks from the baking dish, reserving the marinade in a separate container.

Sprinkle salt and freshly ground black pepper over each lamb rack before cooking.

Toss the lamb shanks in the remaining oil in a large cast-iron pan over medium-high heat for 3-4 minutes, or until they are completely browned on all sides.

Transfer the lamb racks to a serving plate using a slotted spoon.

Continue to cook for about 2 minutes after adding the reserved marinade to the pan.

Set aside to cool gently after removing from the heat.

Place the racks into the pan, meat-side down and bones upright, and cook until the meat is cooked through.

Placing the wok in the oven and baking for approximately 30-40 minutes, basting every 5 minutes with the pan juices, is recommended.

Allow for about 20 minutes before carving after removing the dish from the oven.

To serve, separate the lamb racks and cut them into chops.

Calories and Nutritional Values per Serving

There are 573 calories in this recipe.

33.5% of total calories come from fat. 1.2 g of carbohydrate Sugars: 1.6 g carbohydrate

0.4 g of fiber

0.1 gram of sugar

64 grams of protein

Sodium intake: 201 milligrams

Meatloaf with Veggies Baking Time: 20 minutes Preparation Time Approximately 27 minutes to prepare the dish The following ingredients are used in the preparation of four servings:

8 lamb loin chops (4 ounces each)

12 cup fresh basil leaves (approximate amount)

12-cup sprigs of fresh mint

1 tablespoon of chopped fresh rosemary (or dried rosemary)

2 cloves of garlic

Olive oil (about 3 tblsp. zucchini, sliced into half-moon shapes

1. one large red bell pepper, seeded and cut into large chucks eggplant, sliced into 1 inch pieces

crumbled feta cheese (134 ounces) Cherry tomatoes, 8 ounces

Directions:

390 degrees Fahrenheit should be set as the temperature in your oven.

Fresh herbs, garlic and 2 tablespoons of oil should be combined in a food processor and blended until smooth.

Into a large mixing bowl, add the herb mixture.

In a large mixing bowl, combine the herb mixture and the lamb chops; mix well.

Refrigerate for approximately 2 to 3 hours to allow flavors to blend and blend together.

The zucchini, bell pepper, and eggplant slices should be arranged in the bottom of a large baking sheet, and the remaining oil should be drizzled over them.

Using a single layer of lamb chops, arrange them on the top of the dish.

20 minutes in the oven should suffice.

The chops should be transferred to a serving platter after they have been removed from the oven.

Cover the chops with aluminum foil to keep them warm.

In a separate baking sheet, arrange the cherry tomatoes and sprinkle with the feta cheese. Bake for 20 minutes.

Bake for 5-7 minutes, or until the cheese is just starting to turn golden brown on the edges and edges.

Prepare a vegetable side dish to accompany the chops.

Calories and Nutritional Values per Serving

The following number of calories is 619:

Net Carbohydrates: 9.7 g Fat content: 30.6 g

17.1 g of carbohydrate

7 g fiber 8 g sugar 7 g fiber

69.2 g of protein

331 milligrams of sodium

The Recipes for Beans and Lentils (Chapter 7)

Cooking Time: 15 minutes for the Beans and Veggie Salad. The following ingredients are used in the preparation of four servings:

The following ingredients are needed for the salad:

cooked white beans (approximately three cups)

12 cup black olives, pitted and sliced, 2 medium tomatoes, seeded and chopped 12 cup red onion, chopped

Fresh Italian parsley (chopped finely): 2-3 tablespoons chopped 4-5 sprigs of fresh basil

14 cup extra-virgin olive oil (for dressing).

Red wine vinegar (1-2 tablespoons) grated or minced 1 or 2 garlic cloves

Season with salt and freshly ground black pepper to taste. the bean liquid in three tblsp

Salad preparation instructions: Combine all of the ingredients in a large salad bowl and toss thoroughly.

Mix all of the dressing ingredients together in a separate bowl until thoroughly combined.

Shake the dressing over the salad, making sure it is evenly distributed.

Serve as soon as possible after preparing it. Calories and Nutritional Values per Serving Nutritional Values: 333 Calories

15.7 g of fat; 28.7 g of net carbohydrate 388.8 g of carbohydrate

10.1 g of fiber

2.7 g of sucrose

14 grams of protein

515 milligrams of sodium

Preparation time for the Herbed Beans and Cucumber Salad: 15 minutes. 2 portions per recipe

Ingredients:

The following ingredients are needed for the salad:

a small cucumber that has been finely sliced 2 cups baby arugula (fresh or frozen) 1 small tomato, chopped

1-tablespoon finely chopped fresh parsley a teaspoon of finely minced fresh mint (a 14-ounce can of white navy beans that has been rinsed and drained)

3/3 cup tahini (optional) for dressing

Season with salt and freshly ground black pepper to taste.

tablespoons fresh lemon juice and a 12 teaspoon Aleppo pepper

Salad preparation instructions: Combine all of the ingredients in a large salad bowl and toss thoroughly.

Mix all of the dressing ingredients together in a separate bowl until thoroughly combined.

Shake the dressing over the salad, making sure it is evenly distributed.

Serve as soon as possible after preparing it. Calories and Nutritional Values per Serving There are 398 calories in this recipe.

17.9 g of fat, 25 g of net carbohydrate carbohydrate (43.5 g) fiber (18.5 g) sugar (six g) calories:

18.3 g (g) of protein.

333 milligrams of sodium

Preparation time for Chickpeas and Quinoa Salad: 20 minutes. Approximately 20 minutes for preparation.

Ingredients: 8 servings Nutritional Information:

rinsed and dried 112 cups quinoa 3-cups of distilled water depending on the situation

Extra-virgin olive oil (around 12 cups)

Balsamic vinegar, 1 tablespoon 12 teaspoon dried thyme, crushed 12 teaspoon dried basil, crushed 2 garlic cloves, pressed

peppercorns that have been freshly ground as needed 3 cups arugula (freshly chopped)

1. 1 canned chickpeas (15-ounce can) soaked overnight in water. a third cup pitted and sliced Kalamata olives

a third cup roasted red bell pepper, drained and finely diced 1/4 cup feta cheese, crumbled 1 1/4 cup fresh basil, thinly slivered

Directions:

Pour all of the ingredients into a saucepan and bring to a boil over medium-high heat, stirring frequently.

Low-heat simmering for approximately 20 minutes with the lid on is advised.

Allow for approximately 5 minutes after removing the pan from the heat.

Removing the pan from the heat and setting it aside to cool completely

Dressing preparation: In a large mixing bowl whisk together the olive oil, the vinegar, the garlic, the dried herbs, the salt, and the black pepper until thoroughly combined.

Combine the quinoa, chickpeas, arugula, olives, bell pepper, and feta cheese in a large mixing bowl until everything is well-combined.

Toss the salad with the dressing until it is well coated.

Remove from the oven and garnish with basil before serving! Calories and Nutritional Values per Serving There are 447 calories in this recipe.

19 g (net) of total fat 42.44 g of carbohydrate 57.4 g of carbohydrate

11.9 g of fiber

6.4 g of sucrose

16 grams of protein

1 158 milligrams of sodium

Tomatoes and beans Time required for preparation: 15 minutes 1 14-hour total cooking time The following ingredients are used in the preparation of four servings:

dried lima beans (soaked for 8 hours, then drained) 1 cup 2 sprigs of parsley

1 bouillon cube (vegetable) olive oil (approximately 2-3 tablespoons) minced 2 to 3 garlic cloves

1 / 2 small onion, finely chopped 1 / 2 small carrot, peeled and finely shredded diced tomatoes from a 1512-ounce can one-fourth cup tomato paste

Pure maple syrup (1-2 teaspoons) tablespoons dried oregano 1 teaspoon red wine vinegar 1 teaspoon thyme leaves, dried One-quarter teaspoon of ground nutmeg

Season with salt and freshly ground black pepper to taste. fresh parsley, minced 3 tablespoons fresh mint, minced 3 tablespoons fresh oregano, minced

Directions:

Cook the beans and bay leaf in a large pot of water over high heat until they are tender.

Simmer for approximately 30 minutes on a medium heat setting.

Drain the beans, reserving 1 cup of the cooking liquid in a separate container..

In the hot cooking liquid that has been set aside, dissolve the bouillon cube.

The oven should be set to 375 degrees Fahrenheit.

Sauté the onion and garlic for about 3-4 minutes in a Dutch oven over medium heat until they are soft.

Cook for about 1-2 minutes after you've added the carrot.

Prepare a boiling pot of tomato soup by adding the tomatoes, bouillon cube mixture, and all other ingredients (except for the fresh herbs).

Reduce the heat to a low setting and cook for approximately 10 to 12 minutes longer.

In a separate bowl, mix together the beans, parsley, and mint.

Preheat the oven to 350 degrees for 30-40 minutes after covering the pan with aluminum foil.

Remove the aluminum foil and bake for approximately 10-15 minutes more until the potatoes are tender.

Allow 10 minutes before serving after removing the dish from the oven.

Calories and Nutritional Values per Serving

Amount of calories in this recipe is: 152

7.8 g (net) of total fat 13.7 g of carbohydrates 18.6 g of carbohydrates

4.9 g of fiber

6.4 g of sucrose

4.5 g of protein

170 milligrams of sodium

Beans with Herbs and Spices

15 minutes are required for preparation. Approximately 25 minutes to prepare the dish 4 individual servings

Ingredients:

olive oil (about 2 tbsp.

chopped finely one medium onion (about 1 cup)

Grated fresh ginger (about 12 tablespoon) the finely minced garlic from 2 garlic cloves

12 teaspoon thyme leaves, dried

12 teaspoon oregano leaves (dry), chopped

12 teaspoon dried dill (approximate amount)

ground cumin (about 12 tablespoons)

12 tbsp. coriander leaves, ground chopped finely 1 cup sliced tomatoes 2 cups cannellini beans (in a can or dried)

the broth from 12 cups of vegetables

Season with salt and freshly ground black pepper to taste. freshly chopped parsley (about 2 tablespoons)

Directions: In a large skillet, heat the oil over medium heat and sauté the onion for 6-8 minutes, until softened and translucent.

Cook for approximately 1 minute after adding the ginger, garlic, dried herbs, and spices.

Cook for about 5-6 minutes, crushing the tomatoes with the back of a spoon, until the tomatoes are soft and the sauce is reduced.

In a large mixing bowl, combine the beans and broth.

Cook until it reaches a rolling boil on medium heat.

Simmer for approximately 4-5 minutes, or until the desired consistency is reached, on medium-low heat.

Removing the pan from the heat after seasoning with salt and black pepper

Hot dishes should be garnished with parsley. Calories and Nutritional Values per Serving There are 193 calories in this recipe.

8.5 g of fat per serving 16.6 g of carbohydrate 23.11 g of carbohydrate

6.5 g of fiber

2.54 g sugar; 7.8 g protein; 2.54 g fiber

Sodium is 181 milligrams (mg).

Chapter 5

Lamb Chops with Garlic and Chipotle

Preparation Time: 10 minutes. Approximately 6 minutes of preparation time The following ingredients are used in the preparation of four servings:

Peeled and chopped garlic cloves depending on the situation

1/4 cup crushed, finely ground black mustard seeds ground cumin, 2 teaspoons

ground ginger (one teaspoon)

coriander leaves (ground) 1 teaspoon

12-teaspoon cinnamon powder black peppercorns (to taste) if necessary 8 lamb chops (4 ounces), trimmed and marinated 1 tablespoon extra-virgin olive oil 1 tablespoon lemon juice 1 tablespoon tarragon

Directions:

To prepare the garlic cloves, place them on a cutting board and sprinkle them with a little salt.

Squeeze the garlic until it forms a paste with the help of a knife.

Into a mixing bowl, add the garlic paste.

Mix in the spices and black pepper until everything is evenly distributed.

Slice both sides of the chops with a sharp knife, making 3-4 cuts each time.

Garlic mixture should be generously applied to the chops.

The chops should be cooked for approximately 3 minutes per side in a large cast-iron wok over medium heat.

Serve immediately after drizzling with lemon juice..

Nutritional Information per Serving Calories: 1 g Fat: 0 g Protein: 0 g Fat: 0 g Calories: 0 g 467

20.7% of calories come from fat, and 1.9 grams come from carbohydrate. 2.4 g of carbohydrate

The following nutrients are included: fiber (0.5 g), sugar (0.2 g), and vitamin C.

64.4 g of protein

214 milligrams of sodium

Prepare Lemony Lamb Chops in 10 Minutes Total Time: 10 Minutes Approximately 9 minutes for preparation. 4 individual servings

Ingredients:

Fresh lemon juice and 14 cup extra-virgin olive oil

chopped fresh oregano (about 2 tablespoons) 1 tablespoon minced garlic

Season with salt and freshly ground black pepper to taste. (4) lamb chops (each weighing 8 ounces and 12 inches thick).

Directions:

In a large mixing bowl, combine all of the ingredients except the chops and mix well.

To marinate the chops, place them in a large sealable plastic bag with the marinade.

Stir vigorously to coat everything evenly after sealing the bag.

Allow for about 1 hour of resting time at room temp.

The lamb chops should be removed from the bag and the marinade should be discarded.

To dry the lamb chops, pat them with paper towels.

With a pinch of salt, season the lamb chops.

2 lamb chops should be cooked for about 3 minutes on each side in a large cast-iron grill pan over medium-high heat, if possible.

Cook for approximately 3 more minutes after moving the lamb chops.

Adjust the heat to medium-low after flipping the lamb chops on their sides.

About 2-3 minutes should be sufficient.

Proceed to cook the remainder of the lamb chops in the same fashion.

Removing the lamb chops from the heat and allowing them to rest for approximately 5 minutes before serving

Calories and Nutritional Values per Serving

Nutritional Values: 540 calories

net amount of fat: 29.5 g 0.8 g of carbohydrate 1.8 g of carbohydrate

1 gram of fiber

The amount of sugar in this recipe is 0.3 g

64 grams of protein

213 milligrams of sodium

Rack of Lamb (also known as rack of lamb) is a type of lamb that is roasted on a rack and served with a side of mashed potatoes and vegetables.

15 minutes are required for preparation. Approximately 50 minutes for preparation. 6 portions (per serving)

Ingredients:

extra-virgin olive oil (approximately 12 cup plus 1 tablespoon) crushed garlic cloves (six total)

the leaves of 1 freshly chopped bunch of thyme

1. one bunch of freshly chopped rosemary

1/2 teaspoon red pepper flakes, crushed 2 (112-pound) lamb racks, frenched

Season with salt and freshly ground black pepper to taste.

Directions:

Mix together 12 cup of oil, the garlic, the fresh herbs, and the red pepper flakes in a large baking dish until everything is evenly distributed.

Make a well in the center of the marinade and pour in enough to cover the lamb racks.

Allow at least 6 hours of refrigeration time, flipping once or twice during that time.

Refrigerate for 1 hour before baking on a baking sheet that has been left out at room temperature for that time.

Preheat the oven to 275 degrees Fahrenheit (180 degrees Celsius).

Remove the lamb racks from the baking dish, reserving the marinade in a separate container.

Sprinkle salt and freshly ground black pepper over each lamb rack before cooking.

Toss the lamb shanks in the remaining oil in a large cast-iron pan over medium-high heat for 3-4 minutes, or until they are completely browned on all sides.

Transfer the lamb racks to a serving plate using a slotted spoon.

Continue to cook for about 2 minutes after adding the reserved marinade to the pan.

Set aside to cool gently after removing from the heat.

Place the racks into the pan, meat-side down and bones upright, and cook until the meat is cooked through.

Placing the wok in the oven and baking for approximately 30-40 minutes, basting every 5 minutes with the pan juices, is recommended.

Allow for about 20 minutes before carving after removing the dish from the oven.

To serve, separate the lamb racks and cut them into chops.

Calories and Nutritional Values per Serving

There are 573 calories in this recipe.

33.5% of total calories come from fat. 1.2 g of carbohydrate

Sugars: 1.6 g carbohydrate

0.4 g of fiber

0.1 gram of sugar

64 grams of protein

Sodium intake: 201 milligrams

Meatloaf with Veggies Baking Time: 20 minutes Preparation Time Approximately 27 minutes to prepare the dish The following ingredients are used in the preparation of four servings:

8 lamb loin chops (4 ounces each)

12 cup fresh basil leaves (approximate amount)

12-cup sprigs of fresh mint

1 tablespoon of chopped fresh rosemary (or dried rosemary) 2 cloves of garlic

Olive oil (about 3 tblsp. zucchini, sliced into half-moon shapes

1. one large red bell pepper, seeded and cut into large chucks eggplant, sliced into 1 inch pieces

crumbled feta cheese (134 ounces) Cherry tomatoes, 8 ounces

Directions:

390 degrees Fahrenheit should be set as the temperature in your oven.

Fresh herbs, garlic and 2 tablespoons of oil should be combined in a food processor and blended until smooth.

Into a large mixing bowl, add the herb mixture.

In a large mixing bowl, combine the herb mixture and the lamb chops; mix well.

Refrigerate for approximately 2 to 3 hours to allow flavors to blend and blend together.

The zucchini, bell pepper, and eggplant slices should be arranged in the bottom of a large baking sheet, and the remaining oil should be drizzled over them.

Using a single layer of lamb chops, arrange them on the top of the dish.

20 minutes in the oven should suffice.

The chops should be transferred to a serving platter after they have been removed from the oven.

Cover the chops with aluminum foil to keep them warm.

In a separate baking sheet, arrange the cherry tomatoes and sprinkle with the feta cheese. Bake for 20 minutes.

Bake for 5-7 minutes, or until the cheese is just starting to turn golden brown on the edges and edges.

Prepare a vegetable side dish to accompany the chops.

Calories and Nutritional Values per Serving

The following number of calories is 619:

Net Carbohydrates: 9.7 g Fat content: 30.6 g

17.1 g of carbohydrate

7 g fiber 8 g sugar 7 g fiber

69.2 g of protein

331 milligrams of sodium

The Recipes for Beans and Lentils (Chapter 7)

Cooking Time: 15 minutes for the Beans and Veggie Salad. The following ingredients are used in the preparation of four servings:

The following ingredients are needed for the salad:

cooked white beans (approximately three cups)

12 cup black olives, pitted and sliced, 2 medium tomatoes, seeded and chopped 12 cup red onion, chopped

Fresh Italian parsley (chopped finely): 2-3 tablespoons chopped 4-5 sprigs of fresh basil

14 cup extra-virgin olive oil (for dressing).

Red wine vinegar (1-2 tablespoons) grated or minced 1 or 2 garlic cloves

Season with salt and freshly ground black pepper to taste. the bean liquid in three tblsp

Salad preparation instructions: Combine all of the ingredients in a large salad bowl and toss thoroughly.

Mix all of the dressing ingredients together in a separate bowl until thoroughly combined.

Shake the dressing over the salad, making sure it is evenly distributed.

Serve as soon as possible after preparing it. Calories and Nutritional Values per Serving Nutritional Values: 333 Calories

15.7 g of fat; 28.7 g of net carbohydrate 388.8 g of carbohydrate

10.1 g of fiber

2.7 g of sucrose

14 grams of protein

515 milligrams of sodium

Preparation time for the Herbed Beans and Cucumber Salad: 15 minutes. 2 portions per recipe

Ingredients:

The following ingredients are needed for the salad:

a small cucumber that has been finely sliced 2 cups baby arugula (fresh or frozen) 1 small tomato, chopped

1-tablespoon finely chopped fresh parsley a teaspoon of finely minced fresh mint (a 14-ounce can of white navy beans that has been rinsed and drained)

3/3 cup tahini (optional) for dressing

Season with salt and freshly ground black pepper to taste.

tablespoons fresh lemon juice and a 12 teaspoon Aleppo pepper

Salad preparation instructions: Combine all of the ingredients in a large salad bowl and toss thoroughly.

Mix all of the dressing ingredients together in a separate bowl until thoroughly combined.

Shake the dressing over the salad, making sure it is evenly distributed.

Serve as soon as possible after preparing it. Calories and Nutritional Values per Serving There are 398 calories in this recipe.

17.9 g of fat, 25 g of net carbohydrate carbohydrate (43.5 g) fiber (18.5 g) sugar (six g) calories:

18.3 g (g) of protein.

333 milligrams of sodium

Preparation time for Chickpeas and Quinoa Salad: 20 minutes. Approximately 20 minutes for preparation. Ingredients: 8 servings Nutritional Information:

rinsed and dried 112 cups quinoa 3-cups of distilled water depending on the situation

Extra-virgin olive oil (around 12 cups)

Balsamic vinegar, 1 tablespoon 12 teaspoon dried thyme, crushed 12 teaspoon dried basil, crushed 2 garlic cloves, pressed

peppercorns that have been freshly ground as needed 3 cups arugula (freshly chopped)

1. 1 canned chickpeas (15-ounce can) soaked overnight in water. a third cup pitted and sliced Kalamata olives

a third cup roasted red bell pepper, drained and finely diced 1/4 cup feta cheese, crumbled 1 1/4 cup fresh basil, thinly slivered

Directions:

Pour all of the ingredients into a saucepan and bring to a boil over medium-high heat, stirring frequently.

Low-heat simmering for approximately 20 minutes with the lid on is advised.

Allow for approximately 5 minutes after removing the pan from the heat.

Removing the pan from the heat and setting it aside to cool completely

Dressing preparation: In a large mixing bowl whisk together the olive oil, the vinegar, the garlic, the dried herbs, the salt, and the black pepper until thoroughly combined.

Combine the quinoa, chickpeas, arugula, olives, bell pepper, and feta cheese in a large mixing bowl until everything is well-combined.

Toss the salad with the dressing until it is well coated.

Remove from the oven and garnish with basil before serving! Calories and Nutritional Values per Serving There are 447 calories in this recipe.

19 g (net) of total fat 42.44 g of carbohydrate 57.4 g of carbohydrate

11.9 g of fiber

6.4 g of sucrose

16 grams of protein

1 158 milligrams of sodium

Tomatoes and beans Time required for preparation: 15 minutes 1 14-hour total cooking time The following ingredients are used in the preparation of four servings:

dried lima beans (soaked for 8 hours, then drained) 1 cup 2 sprigs of parsley

1 bouillon cube (vegetable) olive oil (approximately 2-3 tablespoons) minced 2 to 3 garlic cloves

1 / 2 small onion, finely chopped 1 / 2 small carrot, peeled and finely shredded diced tomatoes from a 1512-ounce can one-fourth cup tomato paste

Pure maple syrup (1-2 teaspoons) tablespoons dried oregano 1 teaspoon red wine vinegar 1 teaspoon thyme leaves, dried One-quarter teaspoon of ground nutmeg

Season with salt and freshly ground black pepper to taste. fresh parsley, minced 3 tablespoons fresh mint, minced 3 tablespoons fresh oregano, minced

Directions:

Cook the beans and bay leaf in a large pot of water over high heat until they are tender.

Simmer for approximately 30 minutes on a medium heat setting.

Drain the beans, reserving 1 cup of the cooking liquid in a separate container..

In the hot cooking liquid that has been set aside, dissolve the bouillon cube.

The oven should be set to 375 degrees Fahrenheit.

Sauté the onion and garlic for about 3-4 minutes in a Dutch oven over medium heat until they are soft.

Cook for about 1-2 minutes after you've added the carrot.

Prepare a boiling pot of tomato soup by adding the tomatoes, bouillon cube mixture, and all other ingredients (except for the fresh herbs).

Reduce the heat to a low setting and cook for approximately 10 to 12 minutes longer.

In a separate bowl, mix together the beans, parsley, and mint.

Preheat the oven to 350 degrees for 30-40 minutes after covering the pan with aluminum foil.

Remove the aluminum foil and bake for approximately 10-15 minutes more until the potatoes are tender.

Allow 10 minutes before serving after removing the dish from the oven.

Calories and Nutritional Values per Serving

Amount of calories in this recipe is: 152

7.8 g (net) of total fat 13.7 g of carbohydrates 18.6 g of carbohydrates

4.9 g of fiber

6.4 g of sucrose

4.5 g of protein

170 milligrams of sodium

Beans with Herbs and Spices

15 minutes are required for preparation. Approximately 25 minutes to prepare the dish 4 individual servings

Ingredients:

olive oil (about 2 tbsp.

chopped finely one medium onion (about 1 cup)

Grated fresh ginger (about 12 tablespoon) the finely minced garlic from 2 garlic cloves

12 teaspoon thyme leaves, dried

12 teaspoon oregano leaves (dry), chopped

12 teaspoon dried dill (approximate amount)

ground cumin (about 12 tablespoons)

12 tbsp. coriander leaves, ground chopped finely 1 cup sliced tomatoes 2 cups cannellini beans (in a can or dried)

the broth from 12 cups of vegetables

Season with salt and freshly ground black pepper to taste. freshly chopped parsley (about 2 tablespoons)

Directions: In a large skillet, heat the oil over medium heat and sauté the onion for 6-8 minutes, until softened and translucent.

Cook for approximately 1 minute after adding the ginger, garlic, dried herbs, and spices.

Cook for about 5-6 minutes, crushing the tomatoes with the back of a spoon, until the tomatoes are soft and the sauce is reduced.

In a large mixing bowl, combine the beans and broth.

Cook until it reaches a rolling boil on medium heat.

Simmer for approximately 4-5 minutes, or until the desired consistency is reached, on medium-low heat.

Removing the pan from the heat after seasoning with salt and black pepper

Hot dishes should be garnished with parsley. Calories and Nutritional Values per Serving There are 193 calories in this recipe.

8.5 g of fat per serving 16.6 g of carbohydrate 23.11 g of carbohydrate

6.5 g of fiber

2.54 g sugar; 7.8 g protein; 2.54 g fiber

Sodium is 181 milligrams (mg).

Chapter 6

With Tomato Sauce on the side.

Time Required for Preparation: 20 min Approximately
15 minutes of preparation time Ingredients: 8 servings
Nutritional Information:

lima beans (dried) - 3 cup Water (eight cups):
depending on the situation

Extra-virgin olive oil (14 cup plus 2 tablespoons): 1/2 a
medium-sized yellow onion, finely chopped

1/4 cup finely minced celery stalk (optional) 2 chopped
garlic cloves (peeled) 1 crushed tomato can (28-ounces) dried
oregano (1 teaspoon)

black peppercorns (to taste) if necessary

12-ounce container of crumbled feta cheese 14-ounce
container of fresh parsley

Directions:

Toss the beans with the water and salt in the Instant Pot's pressure cooker.

For 10-12 hours, set aside the pot and allow the beans to soak.

Close the lid and adjust the vent to a position that is completely sealed.

"Manual" is selected, and the cooking time is 15 minutes at "High Pressure".

After the cooking time has expired, select "Cancel" and let the pressure to naturally relax for about 10 minutes before continuing. After then, do a "Quick" release of pressure.

Remove the lid from the pot and drain the beans, reserving 1 cup of the cooking liquid in a separate bowl for later.

The pot should be dried with paper towels.

In an instant pot, add 14 cup of the oil and press "Sauté" to begin cooking. Continue cooking for about 5 minutes after adding the onion, celery, and garlic.

Press "Cancel" and then stir in the beans, the reserved cooking liquid, the tomatoes, the oregano, the salt, and the black pepper until everything is evenly distributed.

Close the lid and adjust the vent to a position that is completely sealed.

Using the default time of 5 minutes, select "Bean/Chili" and press "Start."

After the cooking time has expired, press "Cancel" and allow for a 15-minute "Natural" release to occur. After then, do a "Quick" release of pressure.

Toss the beans mixture into a bowl after opening the lid.

The feta and parsley should be sprinkled on top before serving.

Add the remaining oil and toss to coat the vegetables.

Calories and Nutritional Values per Serving

Nutritional Values: 208 calories

133.3 grams of fat (net) 13.6 g of carbohydrates 18.2 g of carbohydrates

The following nutrients are included: fiber (4.6 grams), sugar (4.7 grams), and protein (6.5 grams).

Amount of sodium in the diet is 144 mg.

Lime Sauced Beans with a Spicy Kick

15 minutes are required for preparation. Approximately 5 minutes of preparation time 1 cup each person; 5 cups total.

Ingredients: jalapenos peppers, finely minced tablespoons freshly squeezed lemon juice 2 chopped garlic cloves 2 fava beans (15 ounces each)

12-cups of liquid

1 teaspoon cumin seeds (ground) depending on the situation olive oil (extra virgin) 1 tablespoon (optional)

12 cup finely chopped fresh parsley (optional). tomato, peeled and diced

Directions:

The sauce is made by combining the jalapenos and garlic in a mortar and pestle and pounding it together.

Remove from heat and stir in the lemon juice.

Put all of the ingredients in a cast-iron pan over medium-high heat and bring to a boil. Remove from heat and set aside to cool.

Using a potato masher, slightly mash the beans once they have been removed from the heat.

In a medium-sized mixing bowl, combine the sauce, oil, and parsley.

Serve with a sprinkling of chopped tomatoes. Calories and Nutritional Values per Serving The following number of calories is 221:

Nutrients: 3 grams of fat, 45.3 grams of carbohydrates, 59.9 g of carbohydrate

Sugar content is 3.8 grams per serving of fiber and 12.5 grams per serving of protein.

Amount of sodium in the diet: 194 mg

Rice Recipes (Chapter 8)

Preparation time for white rice and a veg salad: 15 min. Approximately 20 minutes for preparation. Ingredients: 8 servings Nutritional Information:

water (212 oz)

12 cups long-grain rice, rinsed and drained 12 cups white rice depending on the situation

Extra-virgin olive oil (about a third cup):

Fresh lemon juice (about 14 cups) 2 teaspoons minced fresh oregano 1 garlic clove (peeled and chopped) red pepper flakes (about 1/8 teaspoon) black peppercorns (to taste) if necessary

cups spinach leaves (fresh or frozen) shredded

finely chopped 1 red bell pepper, seeded and sliced

Peel and seed 1 small cucumber, then finely chop the cucumber after it has been seeded.

the following ingredients: 12 cup finely chopped scallion, 12 cup pitted and sliced Kalamata olives, 1 cup of crumbled feta cheese

Directions:

Put the water in a medium-sized saucepan and bring it to a boil over medium heat.

Using a fork, combine the rice and salt.

Simmer, covered, for approximately 15 minutes on a low heat setting.

Set aside for approximately 5 minutes after being removed from heat.

With a fork fluff the rice in the pan after it has been covered.

Set aside to cool somewhat.

For the dressing: in a large bowl, add the oil, lemon juice, garlic, oregano, red pepper flakes, salt, and black pepper and whisk until thoroughly incorporated.

In the bowl of dressing, add the rice and mix to incorporate.

Add the spinach and toss to coat.

Set aside for around 20 minutes.

In the bowl of rice mixture, add the additional ingredients and toss to coat.

Serve as soon as possible after preparing it.

Calories and Nutritional Values per Serving

Calories: 275

Fat: 13.7 g\sNet Carbohydrates: 31.1 g Carbohydrates: 32.7 g

Fiber: 1.6 g

Sugar: 2.5 g

Protein: 6 g

Sodium: 313 mg

Chapter 9: Pasta Recipes

Orzo & Tomato Salad\sPreparation Time: 15 minutes

Cooking Time: 10 minutes 4 individual servings

Ingredients:\sFor Salad

½ cup uncooked whole-wheat orzo pasta 3 plum tomatoes, chopped\s1 cup black olives, pitted and sliced

6 cups fresh spinach, cut approximately 3 onions, chopped\s½ cup feta cheese, crumbled 1 tablespoon capers, drained

For Dressing

1/3 cup olive oil

4 teaspoons fresh lemon juice

1 tablespoon fresh parsley, minced 2 tablespoons fresh lemon zest, grated

Season with salt and freshly ground black pepper to taste.

Directions:

For the salad: in a big pan of the salted boiling water, cook the orzo for around 8-10 minutes or until according to the package directions.

Drain the orzo and rinse under cold running water.

In a large salad bowl, add pasta and additional ingredients and stir. For the dressing: in a small bowl, mix all ingredients and whisk until thoroughly incorporated.

Toss the salad with the dressing until it is well coated.

Refrigerate to cool thoroughly before serving.

Nutritional Information per Serving\sCalories: 340

Fat: 25.1 g\sNet Carbohydrates: 20.8 g Carbohydrates: 25.2 g

Fiber: 4.4 g\sSugar: 4.1 g

Protein: 7.9 g

Sodium: 648 mg

Pasta & Asparagus Salad

15 minutes are required for preparation. Cooking Time: 10 minutes Ingredients: 8 servings Nutritional Information:

1-pound whole-wheat pasta

1-pound fresh asparagus, cut and into bite-sized pieces diagonally 1 tablespoon red wine vinegar

3 teaspoons fresh lemon juice

1-2 teaspoons lemon zest, grated 1 tablespoon olive oil

2-3 cups fresh baby arugula

¼ cup fresh basil, julienned 2/3 cup feta cheese, crumbled\s¼ cup pine nuts, toasted

Freshly cracked black pepper, as necessary

Directions:

In a big pan of the salted water, boil the pasta for approximately 8-10 minutes or until al dente.

In the final 3 minutes of the cooking, mix in the asparagus.

Remove from the heat and pour the pasta and asparagus onto a colander to drain.

Rinse the pasta and asparagus under cold running water and drain thoroughly.

In the same pan, add the asparagus, vinegar, oil, lemon juice, and lemon zest and stir to coat thoroughly.

Add the arugula, basil, feta cheese, pine nuts, and a bit black pepper and gently, toss to coat.

Serve as soon as possible after preparing it. Calories and Nutritional Values per Serving Calories: 298

Fat: 8.7 g\sNet Carbohydrates: 37.2 g Carbohydrates: 44.4 g

Fiber: 7.2 g

Sugar: 3.9 g

Protein: 12 g

Sodium: 197 mg

Pasta & Bell Pepper Salad

15 minutes are required for preparation. Cooking Time: 10 minutes 4 individual servings

Ingredients:

The following ingredients are needed for the salad:

½ cup whole-wheat spiral pasta 1 cup cherry tomatoes, halved 1 cup cucumber, chopped\s½ cup green bell pepper, seeded and cut thinly

½ cup yellow bell pepper, seeded and cut thinly

¼ cup scallion, chopped

2 tablespoons fresh cilantro leaves, chopped\s¼ cup feta cheese, crumbled For Dressing:

olive oil (about 2 tbsp.

lemon juice (about 2 tbsp. fresh) 2 teaspoons water

Season with salt and freshly ground black pepper to taste.

Directions:\sIn a pan of lightly salted boiling water, cook the pasta for approximately 8-10 minutes or according to the package directions.

Drain the pasta thoroughly and leave it aside to cool.

For salad: in a big salad bowl, combine all ingredients except for feta cheese and stir thoroughly.

For dressing: in another small dish, combine all ingredients and whisk thoroughly.

Shake the dressing over the salad, making sure it is evenly distributed.

Set aside at room temperature for approximately 15-20 minutes.

Add pasta and stir to coat thoroughly.

Top with feta and serve immediately. Nutritional Information per Serving Calories: 157

Fat: 9.5 g\sNet Carbohydrates: 13.7 g Carbohydrates: 16.4 g

Fiber: 2.7 g

Sugar: 3.8 g\sProtein: 3.4 g

Sodium: 150 mg

Time Required for Preparation: 15 minutes Pasta, Chicken, and Chickpea Salad Approximately 10 minutes of preparation time The following ingredients are used in this recipe:

The following ingredients are needed for the salad:

penne pasta (about 16 ounces)

cooked chicken breast, thawed and cut into cubes from 2 (161-ounce) boxes cooked chicken breast a can of chickpeas (15 ounces) rinsed and drained (14-ounce) drained and chopped artichoke hearts from a can 12 inch thick rounds of 2 small seedless cucumbers, cut into 1 inch slices 3 bell peppers, seeded and julienned, in various colors

White balsamic vinegar (34 cup) is used for the dressing. garlic cloves (minced) 1 cup olive oil

1 tbsp. Dijon mustard, grated

Season with salt and freshly ground black pepper to taste.

12 cup finely chopped fresh basil (optional).

On top of that, there's a lot to like about this.

7 – 8 ounces crumbled feta cheese

pitted and sliced, a quarter-cup of Kalamata olives

13/14 cup finely chopped fresh basil

Method: Cook the pasta for approximately 8-10 minutes, or according to the package directions, in a large pot of lightly salted boiling water.

The pasta should be thoroughly drained and set aside to cool completely.

To make the salad, combine the pasta with the remaining ingredients in a large salad bowl and toss to combine.

The dressing is made by combining all of the ingredients in a small bowl and mixing thoroughly.

Shake the dressing over the salad, making sure it is evenly distributed.

Place all of the topping ingredients on top of the dish and serve.

Calories and Nutritional Values per Serving

The calories in this recipe are 597 calories.

net amount of fat: 29.5 g 40.10 g of carbohydrate carbohydrate (45.3 g), fiber (5.2 g), protein (1.2 g). 4 g of sucrose

39.1 g of protein

549 milligrams of sodium

Approximately 15 minutes are required for preparation of the pasta and shrimp salad. 8 portions (per serving)

The following ingredients are used in the dressing.

Extra-virgin olive oil (about a third cup):

Fresh lemon juice (around 14 cups)

lemon zest (grated), 1 teaspoon teaspoon of dried oregano a single garlic clove, minced 1 teaspoon paprika rojo (sweet)

Season with salt and freshly ground black pepper to taste.

Salad: 1 cup elbow macaroni that has been cooked

cooked big shrimp weighing 12 ounces cherry tomatoes (cut in half): 2 cups

12 cup red onion, chopped 12 cup Kalamata olives, pitted and sliced 1 green bell pepper, seeded and chopped peeled and pitted avocados (about 2-3) 1 cup finely chopped fresh parsley 1 cup finely chopped fresh mint leaves 4 ounces crumbled feta cheese 1 cup finely chopped fresh parsley

Directions:

Dressing: Combine all of the ingredients in a large mixing bowl until well mixed.

All of the salad ingredients (save the cheese) should be mixed together well in the dressing dish.

Add feta cheese and serve immediately. Calories and Nutritional Values per Serving There are 438 calories in this recipe.

30.4% of the total calories come from fat. 11.8 gram (g) of carbohydrate 29 g of carbohydrates

10.2 g of fiber

4.5 g of sucrose

17 8.8 g (of protein)

400 milligrams of sodium

With Spinach & Tomatoes, Pasta is a delicious option.

15 minutes are required for preparation. Approximately 3 minutes of preparation time 4 individual servings

Ingredients:

Pasta is made using the following ingredients:

Water (four cups)

Spiral pasta (about 10 ounces).

Fresh baby spinach leaves (about 2) quartered 5 cherry tomatoes, a little salt and pepper

2 tablespoons minced garlic, coarsely chopped lemon zest (grated), 1 teaspoon depending on the situation

In order to complete the task:

lemon juice (about 1 tablespoon) olive oil (around 1 tablespoon)

cheese (about 12 cup) ricotta

4 fresh basil leaves chopped 6-8 cherry tomatoes quartered 1/3 cup parmesan cheese, grated 3-4 fresh basil leaves, chopped

2 tablespoons minced garlic, coarsely chopped lemon zest (grated), 1 teaspoon

Season with salt and freshly ground black pepper to taste.

Directions:

To make the pasta, pour all of the ingredients in the instant pot and whisk to incorporate them well..

Close the lid and adjust the vent to a position that is completely sealed.

3 minutes at high pressure with the "Manual" setting selected.

Then, after the cooking time is up, hit "Cancel" and gently push the button labeled "Quick."

After you've opened the cover, whisk in the additional ingredients until everything is properly incorporated.

Serve as soon as possible after preparing it. Calories and Nutritional Values per Serving There are 372 calories in this recipe.

net dietary fat 13.1 g 46.8 g of carbohydrate 46.8 g of carbohydrate

1 gram of fiber

15 g of sugar; 20.5 g of protein

625 milligrams of sodium

Chapter 7

Pasta with artichokes

Pasta with artichokes is a dish that is both delicious and healthy.

15 minutes are required for preparation. Approximately 8 hours of preparation time 4 individual servings

Ingredients:

Cooking spray that is non-stick

Tomatoes with basil, oregano, and garlic in three (1142-ounce) cans 2 artichoke hearts, drained and quartered from a 14-ounce can

1 pound minced garlic cloves

whipping cream (about 12 cup total)

pasta (dried): 12 ounces fettuccine

Green olives with pimiento filling (14 cup)

fourteen-cup (crumbled) feta cheese

Directions:

cooking spray in a large, heavy-bottomed slow cooker

Take two of the canned diced tomatoes and drain the juices.

Toss the drained and undrained tomatoes, along with the artichoke hearts and garlic, into a greased slow cooker and stir until evenly combined.

Set the slow cooker to "Low" and cook, covered, for 6-8 hours on low setting.

During this time, cook the pasta in a large pot of salted boiling water for approximately 8-10 minutes, or according to package directions.

Under cold running water, drain the pasta and rinse it.

Uncover the slow cooker and gently stir in the heavy whipping cream once the cooking time is completed.

Pasta should be divided between serving plates and topped with artichoke sauce.

Finish by garnishing with olives and cheese and serving it immediately.

Calories and Nutritional Values per Serving

Nutritional Values: 479 Calories

10.4 g (net) of total fat 67.4 g of carbohydrate 80.22 g of carbohydrate

14.8 g of fiber

10.5 g of sucrose

20.8 g of protein

407 milligrams of sodium

Soup and Stew Recipes (Chapter 10)

Preparation Time for Yellow Squash Soup: 15 min. Approximately 35 minutes for preparation. 6 portions (per serving)

Ingredients:

unsalted butter (approximately 2 tablespoons) 3 large green peppers, peeled and chopped 6 garlic cloves, minced

yellow squash, seeded and cubed (about 6 cups total) 4 sprigs of fresh thyme

broth (vegetable) (4 cups)

Season with salt and freshly ground black pepper to taste. lemon juice (about 2 tbsp. fresh)

4 tablespoons of shredded Parmesan cheese freshly grated lemon peel (about 2 teaspoons)

Directions:

The onions should be sautéed for about 5-6 minutes in a large soup pan with the butter on medium heat.

Cook for about 1 minute after adding the garlic.

Cook for about 5 minutes after you've added the yellow squash cubes.

Bring the broth, thyme, salt, and black pepper to a boil, stirring constantly.

Low-heat cooking for approximately 15-20 minutes with the lid on is recommended.

After removing the pan from the heat, discard the thyme sprigs and set it aside.

Remove the pan from the heat and set it aside to cool a bit.

Mixing in batches in a large blender will help to ensure that the soup is smooth.

Return the soup to the same pan and heat it over medium heat until it has thickened slightly again.

Cook for approximately 2-3 minutes, or until the lemon juice has been completely absorbed by the sauce.

Remove from the oven and top with the cheese and lemon peel before serving immediately.

Calories and Nutritional Values per Serving

Nutritional Values: 115 calories

6 g (net) fat 7.3 g of carbohydrates 9.8 g of carbohydrate

2.5 g of fiber

4.2 g of sucrose

6.6 g of protein

634 milligrams of sodium

The preparation time for this soup is 15 minutes. Approximately 40 minutes for preparation. 1 cup each person; 5 cups total.

Ingredients:

1 cup extra-virgin olive oil 2 tablespoons adobo 4 medium carrots, peeled and chopped 2 celery stalks, peeled and chopped 1 large red onion, peeled and chopped two crushed garlic cloves, a dozen pounds of fresh kale (with tough ribs removed and chopped), and a pinch of salt 36.12 quarts of chicken stock

Season with salt and freshly ground black pepper to taste.

Directions:

Cook the carrots, celery, onion, and garlic for about 8-10 minutes, stirring frequently, in a large soup pan coated with oil over medium heat.

Cook for 5 minutes, stirring twice, until the kale is tender.

Boil the broth after you've added the rest of your ingredients.

Cook for about 20 minutes with the lid partially open.

Remove from the heat and season with salt and black pepper.

Blend the soup until it is smooth using an immersion blender.

Serve as soon as possible after preparing it. Calories and Nutritional Values per Serving Nutritional information per serving: 140 calories

Carbohydrates (net): 11.1 g, 6.9 g fat 13.8 g of carbohydrates

2.7 g of fiber, 4.4 g of sugar

2.6 g of protein

15 minutes to prepare Potato and Broccoli Soup with 778 mg of sodium 6 Minutes Preparation Time Ingredients: 4 tablespoons extra-virgin olive oil Servings: 4

medium onion, chopped finely 1 large celery stalk, chopped 1 large carrot, chopped medium white potatoes, peeled and cubed 2 large garlic cloves, chopped 4 cups vegetable broth 1 pound broccoli chopped medium white potatoes, peeled and cubed

Season with salt and freshly ground black pepper to taste.

12 cup heavy cream made from coconut

lemon juice (fresh squeezed) 1 teaspoon

fresh parsley, chopped (about 2 tablespoons total)

Sauté the oil in the instant pot according to the manufacturer's instructions. Continue cooking for 3-4 minutes after adding the celery and onion.

After pressing "Cancel," combine the remaining ingredients, minus the lemon juice, in a large mixing bowl.

Close the lid and adjust the vent to a position that is completely sealed.

3 minutes at high pressure with the "Manual" setting selected.

Immediately after the cooking time has expired, press "Cancel" and perform a 5-minute "Natural" release. After then, do a "Quick" release of pressure.

Remove the lid and blend the soup until it is smooth using an immersion blender.

Serve immediately with a dollop of coconut cream and a squeeze of lemon juice for garnish.

Calories and Nutritional Values per Serving

Nutritional Values: 294 calories

16.1 g of fat, 23.2 g of net carbohydrate 30.11 gram of carbohydrate

The following nutrients are found in this serving: Fiber: 6.9 g Sugar: 6.2 g

11 grams of protein

the following amounts of sodium: 856 mg

Approximately 15 minutes to prepare Split Pea Soup

Approximately 15 minutes of preparation time Recipe serves 6 people; ingredients are as follows.

olive oil (11,2 tablespoons)

Peel and chop 1 medium carrot (approximately) 4 celery stalks, finely chopped 1 medium white onion, chopped 1 celery stalk, finely chopped 5 garlic cloves, finely chopped

rinsed and drained two cups yellow split peas

12 cup diced tomatoes from a tin can 2 sprigs of parsley

1-tsp. paprika, to taste

ground cumin (11 2 teaspoons)

1 / 4 teaspoon cinnamon powder

cayenne pepper (14 teaspoon) depending on the situation

vegetable broth (about 7 cups)

lemon juice (about 1 tablespoon)

Greek yogurt (plain) (12 cup)

Directions:

In an instant pot, combine the oil and the "Sauté" setting. Continue cooking for about 4 minutes after adding the carrot and onion.

Cook for about 1 minute after you add the garlic!

Press "Cancel" and stir in the rest of the ingredients, excluding the lemon juice and the yogurt, until everything is well combined.

Close the lid and adjust the vent to a position that is completely sealed.

Cook for 10 minutes at "High Pressure" on the "Manual" setting.

After the cooking time has expired, select "Cancel" and let the pressure to naturally relax for about 10 minutes before continuing. After then, do a "Quick" release of pressure.

Toss in the lemon juice after opening the lid.

Place yogurt on top of the dish and serve immediately. Calories and Nutritional Values per Serving There are 245 calories in this recipe.

Net dietary fat: 5 g 21 g carbohydrate Carbohydrates: 35.7 g carbohydrates 13.6 g of fiber

7.1 g of sucrose

18.4 g of protein

717 milligrams of sodium

Cooking Soup with Beans and Wild Rice

15 minutes are required for preparation. Approximately 50 minutes for preparation. Recipe serves 6 people; ingredients are as follows.

8 cups vegetable broth (distributed evenly). wild rice, drained and rinsed 1 cup

2 carrots, peeled and chopped 4 celery stalks, chopped 1 cup carrots, chopped 12 onions, chopped

1 onion, peeled and sliced 1-teaspoon thyme leaves dried bay leaves (approximately 2)

depending on the situation

1. Cannellini beans, rinsed and drained from a 15-ounce can. raw cashews, soaked overnight and drained; 8 ounces, finely chopped fresh mushrooms.

Cooking Instructions: In a large saucepan, combine 7 cups broth and bring to a boil over medium-high heat.

Again, bring the pot to a boil, and add the wild rice, celery, carrots (if using), onion, garlic (if using), thyme, bay leaves, and salt.

Cook for approximately 30 minutes with the lid on the pan.

The beans, cashews, and remaining broth should be blended together on high speed until completely smooth in the meantime.

Stir in the beans and mushrooms until everything is well combined.

Simmer, covered, for approximately 15 minutes on a low heat setting.

The bay leaves should be discarded after removing the dish from the heat.

Hot food should be served.

Calories in a serving: 394 Calories in one serving

The following are the macronutrients: fat (12.9 g), net carbohydrates (36.5 g), and protein. 46.33 g of carbohydrate

6.8 g of fiber

4.2 g of sucrose

29.4 g of protein

Eleven hundred sixty-three grams of sodium

Chapter 8

Pasta e Fagioli Soup

Cooking Time: 15 minutes for Pasta e Fagioli Soup. Approximately 27 minutes to prepare the dish 8 portions (per serving)

Tablespoon extra-virgin olive oil Ingredients:
thinly sliced celery stalks (or celery leaves)
Peeled and chopped carrots (about 2 cups) 1/2 of a large yellow onion, finely minced
minced 4 garlic cloves (peeled and peeled), the ground beef was 112 pounds 2 teaspoons chili powder (or equivalent)
diced tomatoes (1 1412-ounce can)
great northern white beans, rinsed and drained (one 15-ounce can total). red kidney beans, rinsed and drained from one (15-ounce) can.
macaroni (elbow) 5 ounces, uncooked 1 tomato sauce can (approximately 1412 ounces).
chicken broth (about 5 cups)

Season with salt and freshly ground black pepper to taste.

Grated 12 cup Parmigiano-Reggiano

Directions:

In an instant pot, combine the oil and the "Sauté" setting. Continue to cook for about 4-5 minutes after you've added the carrots and celery.

Cook for about 1 minute after you add the garlic!

Cook for about 6-8 minutes after adding the ground beef.

Remove the pot from the heat and drain any remaining grease.

Cook for about 1 minute after adding the chili powder.

Cook for approximately 6 to 8 minutes after adding the tomato puree to the pan.

Toss in the beans, pasta, tomato sauce, and broth after pressing "Cancel."

Close the lid and adjust the vent to a position that is completely sealed.

"Manual" is selected, and the cooking time is 4 minutes at "High Pressure."

Immediately after the cooking time has expired, press "Cancel" and perform a 5-minute "Natural" release. After then, do a "Quick" release of pressure.

To serve, remove the lid and top with cheese.

Calories and Nutritional Values per Serving

There are 448 calories in a serving.

10 g fat, 34.5 g carbohydrate (net), 1 g protein 46.33 g of carbohydrate

11.8 g of fiber

7.9 g of sucrose

42 grams of protein

the amount of sodium in 963 milligrams

Soup made with lentils and vegetables

15 minutes are required for preparation. Approximately 45 minutes for preparation. The following ingredients are used in the preparation of four servings:

coconut oil (one tablespoon)

Peeled and chopped medium-sized carrots one-half cup finely chopped white onion

minced 4 garlic cloves (peeled and peeled),

freshly minced ginger (about 1 teaspoon total)

Season with salt and freshly ground black pepper to taste. Sweet potatoes, peeled and cubed (about 3 cups total). curry powder (11 1/2 tablespoons)

vegetable broth (approximately 5-6 cups).

one-half cup cooked green lentils (rinsed and drained). fresh baby spinach (about 4 cups)

tablespoon coconut sugar tablespoons freshly squeezed lemon juice (optional)

The carrots, onion, garlic, and ginger should be sautéed for about 3-5 minutes in a large pan with the oil heated over medium heat.

Cook for 3-4 minutes, stirring occasionally, until the sweet potatoes are soft.

Cook for about 2 minutes after adding the curry powder.

In a large mixing bowl, combine the lentils and broth.

Cook until it reaches a rolling boil on medium heat.

Cook for about 20-25 minutes, uncovered, on low heat, until the lentils and potatoes are tender, about 20-25 minutes.

Cook for approximately 3-5 minutes after adding the kale and coconut sugar.

Removing it from the heat after stirring in the lemon juice

Hot food should be served.

Calories and Nutritional Values per Serving

Nutrients: 455 calories

4.5 g of fat per serving 67.1 g of carbohydrates 89.6 g of carbohydrates

22.5% of calories come from fiber, and 14.6 percent come from sugar.

17.2 g of protein

554 milligrams of sodium

Vegan and vegetarian recipes are covered in Chapter 11.

Cooking Time: 10 minutes for the Orange & Kale Salad Recipe serves 2 people; ingredients are as follows.

kale, tough ribs removed and torn into small pieces for salad cups. peeled and cut into segments: 2 oranges

1 cup dried cranberries, chopped

Dressings are made with:

olive oil (about 2 tbsp.

freshly squeezed orange juice (about 2 tablespoons)

sugar substitute (12 teaspoon agave nectar). depending on the situation

Directions:

Mix all of the ingredients together in a salad bowl before serving.

Using a separate bowl, combine all of the dressing ingredients and whisk until well blended.

Shake the dressing over the salad, making sure it is well distributed.

Serve as soon as possible after preparing it. Serving Size and Nutritional Information Calories: 273 per serving

net dietary fat 14.3 g Carbon dioxide: 29.4 g Carbohydrates: 35.7 g Carbon dioxide: 29.5 g

6.3 g of fiber

The following are the nutritional values for this dish: sugar (20 g); protein (4.8 g).

Sodium intake: 121 milligrams

Snack Recipes (Chapter 12):

Pumkin Seeds (Roasted)

Approximately 10 minutes are required for preparation. Approximately 20 minutes for preparation. 4 individual servings

Ingredients:

34 cup pumpkin seeds, soaked in water and then dried red chili powder (one-third teaspoon)

ground turmeric (14 teaspoon) depending on the situation

coconut oil (melted) (3 tablespoons)

Fresh lemon juice (approximately 12 tablespoons)

Directions:

350 degrees Fahrenheit (180 degrees Celsius) Preheat the oven.

Stir well to coat everything with oil and vinegar (except the lemon juice).

A baking sheet should be used to transfer the pumpkin seed mixture.

Turning once or twice during cooking time will ensure even browning.

Allow to cool completely before serving. Remove from oven and set aside.

Serve with a squeeze of fresh lemon juice. Calories and Nutritional Values per Serving There are 276 calories in a serving.

26.11 g (net) of total fat 4.9 g of carbohydrate 6.4 g of carbohydrate

Nutritional Values: 1.5 grams of fiber, 0.4grams of sugar, 8.6 grams of protein.

Amount of sodium in one serving: 69 mg

Almonds (Roasted)

Minutes required for preparation: 5 Approximately 10 minutes of preparation time 4 individual servings

Ingredients:

Whole almonds (about 1 cup total)

12-teaspoon cinnamon powder

ground cumin, 14 teaspoon

Season with salt and freshly ground black pepper to taste. olive oil (about 2 tbsp.

Directions:

Place parchment paper in the bottom of a baking dish.

Into a large mixing bowl, combine all of the ingredients and thoroughly combine.

A single layer of almonds should be spread out into a baking dish that has been prepared in advance of baking.

Turning twice during the roasting process.

Remove the almonds from the oven and set them aside to cool completely before serving them up.

Calories and Nutritional Values per Serving

Calories in a serving (198 calories)

18 g (net) of fat 2.2 g of carbohydrate 5.3 g of carbohydrate 3.1 g of fiber

The sugar content is one gram, and the protein content is four grams.

42 mg of sodiumTime Required for Preparation: 15 minutes Pasta, Chicken, and Chickpea Salad Approximately 10 minutes

of preparation time The following ingredients are used in this recipe:

The following ingredients are needed for the salad:

penne pasta (about 16 ounces)

cooked chicken breast, thawed and cut into cubes from 2 (161-ounce) boxes cooked chicken breast a can of chickpeas (15 ounces) rinsed and drained (14-ounce) drained and chopped artichoke hearts from a can 12 inch thick rounds of 2 small seedless cucumbers, cut into 1 inch slices 3 bell peppers, seeded and julienned, in various colors

White balsamic vinegar (34 cup) is used for the dressing. garlic cloves (minced) 1 cup olive oil

1 tbsp. Dijon mustard, grated

Season with salt and freshly ground black pepper to taste.

12 cup finely chopped fresh basil (optional).

On top of that, there's a lot to like about this.

7 – 8 ounces crumbled feta cheese

pitted and sliced, a quarter-cup of Kalamata olives

13/14 cup finely chopped fresh basil

Method: Cook the pasta for approximately 8-10 minutes, or according to the package directions, in a large pot of lightly salted boiling water.

The pasta should be thoroughly drained and set aside to cool completely.

To make the salad, combine the pasta with the remaining ingredients in a large salad bowl and toss to combine.

The dressing is made by combining all of the ingredients in a small bowl and mixing thoroughly.

Shake the dressing over the salad, making sure it is evenly distributed.

Place all of the topping ingredients on top of the dish and serve.

Calories and Nutritional Values per Serving

The calories in this recipe are 597 calories.

net amount of fat: 29.5 g 40.10 g of carbohydrate carbohydrate (45.3 g), fiber (5.2 g), protein (1.2 g). 4 g of sucrose

39.1 g of protein

549 milligrams of sodium

Approximately 15 minutes are required for preparation of the pasta and shrimp salad. 8 portions (per serving)

The following ingredients are used in the dressing.

Extra-virgin olive oil (about a third cup):

Fresh lemon juice (around 14 cups)

lemon zest (grated), 1 teaspoon teaspoon of dried oregano a single garlic clove, minced 1 teaspoon paprika rojo (sweet)

Season with salt and freshly ground black pepper to taste.

Salad: 1 cup elbow macaroni that has been cooked

cooked big shrimp weighing 12 ounces cherry tomatoes (cut in half): 2 cups

12 cup red onion, chopped 12 cup Kalamata olives, pitted and sliced 1 green bell pepper, seeded and chopped peeled and

pitted avocados (about 2-3) 1 cup finely chopped fresh parsley 1 cup finely chopped fresh mint leaves 4 ounces crumbled feta cheese 1 cup finely chopped fresh parsley

Directions:

Dressing: Combine all of the ingredients in a large mixing bowl until well mixed.

All of the salad ingredients (save the cheese) should be mixed together well in the dressing dish.

Add feta cheese and serve immediately. Calories and Nutritional Values per Serving There are 438 calories in this recipe.

30.4% of the total calories come from fat. 11.8 gram (g) of carbohydrate 29 g of carbohydrates

10.2 g of fiber

4.5 g of sucrose

17 8.8 g (of protein)

400 milligrams of sodium

With Spinach & Tomatoes, Pasta is a delicious option.

15 minutes are required for preparation. Approximately 3 minutes of preparation time 4 individual servings

Ingredients:

Pasta is made using the following ingredients:

Water (four cups)

Spiral pasta (about 10 ounces).

Fresh baby spinach leaves (about 2) quartered 5 cherry tomatoes, a little salt and pepper

2 tablespoons minced garlic, coarsely chopped lemon zest (grated), 1 teaspoon depending on the situation

In order to complete the task:

lemon juice (about 1 tablespoon) olive oil (around 1 tablespoon)

cheese (about 12 cup) ricotta

4 fresh basil leaves chopped 6-8 cherry tomatoes quartered 1/3 cup parmesan cheese, grated 3-4 fresh basil leaves, chopped

2 tablespoons minced garlic, coarsely chopped lemon zest (grated), 1 teaspoon

Season with salt and freshly ground black pepper to taste.

Directions:

To make the pasta, pour all of the ingredients in the instant pot and whisk to incorporate them well..

Close the lid and adjust the vent to a position that is completely sealed.

3 minutes at high pressure with the "Manual" setting selected.

Then, after the cooking time is up, hit "Cancel" and gently push the button labeled "Quick."

After you've opened the cover, whisk in the additional ingredients until everything is properly incorporated.

Serve as soon as possible after preparing it. Calories and Nutritional Values per Serving There are 372 calories in this recipe.

net dietary fat 13.1 g 46.8 g of carbohydrate 46.8 g of carbohydrate

1 gram of fiber

15 g of sugar; 20.5 g of protein

625 milligrams of sodium

Pasta with artichokes is a dish that is both delicious and healthy.

15 minutes are required for preparation. Approximately 8 hours of preparation time 4 individual servings

Ingredients:

Cooking spray that is non-stick

Tomatoes with basil, oregano, and garlic in three (1142-ounce) cans 2 artichoke hearts, drained and quartered from a 14-ounce can

1 pound minced garlic cloves

whipping cream (about 12 cup total)

pasta (dried): 12 ounces fettuccine

Green olives with pimiento filling (14 cup)

fourteen-cup (crumbled) feta cheese

Directions:

cooking spray in a large, heavy-bottomed slow cooker

Take two of the canned diced tomatoes and drain the juices.

Toss the drained and undrained tomatoes, along with the artichoke hearts and garlic, into a greased slow cooker and stir until evenly combined.

Set the slow cooker to "Low" and cook, covered, for 6-8 hours on low setting.

During this time, cook the pasta in a large pot of salted boiling water for approximately 8-10 minutes, or according to package directions.

Under cold running water, drain the pasta and rinse it.

Uncover the slow cooker and gently stir in the heavy whipping cream once the cooking time is completed.

Pasta should be divided between serving plates and topped with artichoke sauce.

Finish by garnishing with olives and cheese and serving it immediately.

Calories and Nutritional Values per Serving

Nutritional Values: 479 Calories

10.4 g (net) of total fat 67.4 g of carbohydrate 80.22 g of carbohydrate

14.8 g of fiber

10.5 g of sucrose

20.8 g of protein

407 milligrams of sodium

Chapter 9

Soup and Stew Recipes

Preparation Time for Yellow Squash Soup: 15 min. Approximately 35 minutes for preparation. 6 portions (per serving)

Ingredients:

unsalted butter (approximately 2 tablespoons) 3 large green peppers, peeled and chopped 6 garlic cloves, minced

yellow squash, seeded and cubed (about 6 cups total) 4 sprigs of fresh thyme

broth (vegetable) (4 cups)

Season with salt and freshly ground black pepper to taste. lemon juice (about 2 tbsp. fresh)

4 tablespoons of shredded Parmesan cheese freshly grated lemon peel (about 2 teaspoons)

Directions:

The onions should be sautéed for about 5-6 minutes in a large soup pan with the butter on medium heat.

Cook for about 1 minute after adding the garlic.

Cook for about 5 minutes after you've added the yellow squash cubes.

Bring the broth, thyme, salt, and black pepper to a boil, stirring constantly.

Low-heat cooking for approximately 15-20 minutes with the lid on is recommended.

After removing the pan from the heat, discard the thyme sprigs and set it aside.

Remove the pan from the heat and set it aside to cool a bit.

Mixing in batches in a large blender will help to ensure that the soup is smooth.

Return the soup to the same pan and heat it over medium heat until it has thickened slightly again.

Cook for approximately 2-3 minutes, or until the lemon juice has been completely absorbed by the sauce.

Remove from the oven and top with the cheese and lemon peel before serving immediately.

Calories and Nutritional Values per Serving

Nutritional Values: 115 calories

6 g (net) fat 7.3 g of carbohydrates 9.8 g of carbohydrate

2.5 g of fiber

4.2 g of sucrose

6.6 g of protein

634 milligrams of sodium

The preparation time for this soup is 15 minutes. Approximately 40 minutes for preparation. 1 cup each person; 5 cups total.

Ingredients:

1 cup extra-virgin olive oil 2 tablespoons adobo 4 medium carrots, peeled and chopped 2 celery stalks, peeled and chopped 1 large red onion, peeled and chopped two crushed garlic cloves, a dozen pounds of fresh kale (with tough ribs removed and chopped), and a pinch of salt 36.12 quarts of chicken stock

Season with salt and freshly ground black pepper to taste.

Directions:

Cook the carrots, celery, onion, and garlic for about 8-10 minutes, stirring frequently, in a large soup pan coated with oil over medium heat.

Cook for 5 minutes, stirring twice, until the kale is tender.

Boil the broth after you've added the rest of your ingredients.

Cook for about 20 minutes with the lid partially open.

Remove from the heat and season with salt and black pepper.

Blend the soup until it is smooth using an immersion blender.

Serve as soon as possible after preparing it. Calories and Nutritional Values per Serving Nutritional information per serving: 140 calories

Carbohydrates (net): 11.1 g, 6.9 g fat 13.8 g of carbohydrates

2.7 g of fiber, 4.4 g of sugar

2.6 g of protein

15 minutes to prepare Potato and Broccoli Soup with 778 mg of sodium 6 Minutes Preparation Time Ingredients: 4 tablespoons extra-virgin olive oil Servings: 4

medium onion, chopped finely 1 large celery stalk, chopped 1 large carrot, chopped medium white potatoes, peeled and cubed 2 large garlic cloves, chopped 4 cups vegetable broth 1 pound broccoli chopped medium white potatoes, peeled and cubed

Season with salt and freshly ground black pepper to taste.

12 cup heavy cream made from coconut

lemon juice (fresh squeezed) 1 teaspoon

fresh parsley, chopped (about 2 tablespoons total)

Sauté the oil in the instant pot according to the manufacturer's instructions. Continue cooking for 3-4 minutes after adding the celery and onion.

After pressing "Cancel," combine the remaining ingredients, minus the lemon juice, in a large mixing bowl.

Close the lid and adjust the vent to a position that is completely sealed.

3 minutes at high pressure with the "Manual" setting selected.

Immediately after the cooking time has expired, press "Cancel" and perform a 5-minute "Natural" release. After then, do a "Quick" release of pressure.

Remove the lid and blend the soup until it is smooth using an immersion blender.

Serve immediately with a dollop of coconut cream and a squeeze of lemon juice for garnish.

Calories and Nutritional Values per Serving

Nutritional Values: 294 calories

16.1 g of fat, 23.2 g of net carbohydrate 30.11 gram of carbohydrate

The following nutrients are found in this serving: Fiber: 6.9 g Sugar: 6.2 g

11 grams of protein

the following amounts of sodium: 856 mg

Approximately 15 minutes to prepare Split Pea Soup Approximately 15 minutes of preparation time Recipe serves 6 people; ingredients are as follows.

olive oil (11,2 tablespoons)

Peel and chop 1 medium carrot (approximately) 4 celery stalks, finely chopped 1 medium white onion, chopped 1 celery stalk, finely chopped 5 garlic cloves, finely chopped

rinsed and drained two cups yellow split peas

12 cup diced tomatoes from a tin can 2 sprigs of parsley

1-tsp. paprika, to taste

ground cumin (11 2 teaspoons)

1 / 4 teaspoon cinnamon powder

cayenne pepper (14 teaspoon) depending on the situation

vegetable broth (about 7 cups)

lemon juice (about 1 tablespoon)

Greek yogurt (plain) (12 cup)

Directions:

In an instant pot, combine the oil and the "Sauté" setting. Continue cooking for about 4 minutes after adding the carrot and onion.

Cook for about 1 minute after you add the garlic!

Press "Cancel" and stir in the rest of the ingredients, excluding the lemon juice and the yogurt, until everything is well combined.

Close the lid and adjust the vent to a position that is completely sealed.

Cook for 10 minutes at "High Pressure" on the "Manual" setting.

After the cooking time has expired, select "Cancel" and let the pressure to naturally relax for about 10 minutes before continuing. After then, do a "Quick" release of pressure.

Toss in the lemon juice after opening the lid.

Place yogurt on top of the dish and serve immediately. Calories and Nutritional Values per Serving There are 245 calories in this recipe.

Net dietary fat: 5 g 21 g carbohydrate Carbohydrates: 35.7 g carbohydrates 13.6 g of fiber

7.1 g of sucrose

18.4 g of protein

717 milligrams of sodium

Cooking Soup with Beans and Wild Rice

15 minutes are required for preparation. Approximately 50 minutes for preparation. Recipe serves 6 people; ingredients are as follows.

8 cups vegetable broth (distributed evenly). wild rice, drained and rinsed 1 cup

2 carrots, peeled and chopped 4 celery stalks, chopped 1 cup carrots, chopped 12 onions, chopped

1 onion, peeled and sliced 1-teaspoon thyme leaves dried bay leaves (approximately 2)

depending on the situation

1. Cannellini beans, rinsed and drained from a 15-ounce can. raw cashews, soaked overnight and drained; 8 ounces, finely chopped fresh mushrooms.

Cooking Instructions: In a large saucepan, combine 7 cups broth and bring to a boil over medium-high heat.

Again, bring the pot to a boil, and add the wild rice, celery, carrots (if using), onion, garlic (if using), thyme, bay leaves, and salt.

Cook for approximately 30 minutes with the lid on the pan.

The beans, cashews, and remaining broth should be blended together on high speed until completely smooth in the meantime.

Stir in the beans and mushrooms until everything is well combined.

Simmer, covered, for approximately 15 minutes on a low heat setting.

The bay leaves should be discarded after removing the dish from the heat.

Hot food should be served.

Calories in a serving: 394 Calories in one serving

The following are the macronutrients: fat (12.9 g), net carbohydrates (36.5 g), and protein. 46.33 g of carbohydrate

6.8 g of fiber

4.2 g of sucrose

29.4 g of protein

Eleven hundred sixty-three grams of sodium

Cooking Time: 15 minutes for Pasta e Fagioli Soup. Approximately 27 minutes to prepare the dish 8 portions (per serving)

Tablespoon extra-virgin olive oil Ingredients:

thinly sliced celery stalks (or celery leaves)

Peeled and chopped carrots (about 2 cups) 1/2 of a large yellow onion, finely minced

minced 4 garlic cloves (peeled and peeled), the ground beef was 112 pounds 2 teaspoons chili powder (or equivalent)

diced tomatoes (1 1412-ounce can)

great northern white beans, rinsed and drained (one 15-ounce can total). red kidney beans, rinsed and drained from one (15-ounce) can.

macaroni (elbow) 5 ounces, uncooked 1 tomato sauce can (approximately 1412 ounces).

chicken broth (about 5 cups)

Season with salt and freshly ground black pepper to taste.

Grated 12 cup Parmigiano-Reggiano

Directions:

In an instant pot, combine the oil and the "Sauté" setting. Continue to cook for about 4-5 minutes after you've added the carrots and celery.

Cook for about 1 minute after you add the garlic!

Cook for about 6-8 minutes after adding the ground beef.

Remove the pot from the heat and drain any remaining grease.

Cook for about 1 minute after adding the chili powder.

Cook for approximately 6 to 8 minutes after adding the tomato puree to the pan.

Toss in the beans, pasta, tomato sauce, and broth after pressing "Cancel."

Close the lid and adjust the vent to a position that is completely sealed.

"Manual" is selected, and the cooking time is 4 minutes at "High Pressure."

Immediately after the cooking time has expired, press "Cancel" and perform a 5-minute "Natural" release. After then, do a "Quick" release of pressure.

To serve, remove the lid and top with cheese.

Calories and Nutritional Values per Serving

There are 448 calories in a serving.

10 g fat, 34.5 g carbohydrate (net), 1 g protein 46.33 g of carbohydrate

11.8 g of fiber

7.9 g of sucrose

42 grams of protein

the amount of sodium in 963 milligrams

Soup made with lentils and vegetables

15 minutes are required for preparation. Approximately 45 minutes for preparation. The following ingredients are used in the preparation of four servings:

coconut oil (one tablespoon)

Peeled and chopped medium-sized carrots one-half cup finely chopped white onion

minced 4 garlic cloves (peeled and peeled),

freshly minced ginger (about 1 teaspoon total)

Season with salt and freshly ground black pepper to taste. Sweet potatoes, peeled and cubed (about 3 cups total). curry powder (11 1/2 tablespoons)

vegetable broth (approximately 5-6 cups).

one-half cup cooked green lentils (rinsed and drained). fresh baby spinach (about 4 cups)

tablespoon coconut sugar tablespoons freshly squeezed lemon juice (optional)

The carrots, onion, garlic, and ginger should be sautéed for about 3-5 minutes in a large pan with the oil heated over medium heat.

Cook for 3-4 minutes, stirring occasionally, until the sweet potatoes are soft.

Cook for about 2 minutes after adding the curry powder.

In a large mixing bowl, combine the lentils and broth.

Cook until it reaches a rolling boil on medium heat.

Cook for about 20-25 minutes, uncovered, on low heat, until the lentils and potatoes are tender, about 20-25 minutes.

Cook for approximately 3-5 minutes after adding the kale and coconut sugar.

Removing it from the heat after stirring in the lemon juice

Hot food should be served.

Calories and Nutritional Values per Serving

Nutrients: 455 calories

4.5 g of fat per serving 67.1 g of carbohydrates 89.6 g of carbohydrates

22.5% of calories come from fiber, and 14.6 percent come from sugar.

17.2 g of protein

554 milligrams of sodium

Vegan and vegetarian recipes are covered in Chapter 11.

Cooking Time: 10 minutes for the Orange & Kale Salad Recipe serves 2 people; ingredients are as follows.

kale, tough ribs removed and torn into small pieces for salad cups. peeled and cut into segments: 2 oranges

1 cup dried cranberries, chopped

Dressings are made with:

olive oil (about 2 tbsp.

freshly squeezed orange juice (about 2 tablespoons)

sugar substitute (12 teaspoon agave nectar). depending on the situation

Directions:

Mix all of the ingredients together in a salad bowl before serving.

Using a separate bowl, combine all of the dressing ingredients and whisk until well blended.

Shake the dressing over the salad, making sure it is well distributed.

Serve as soon as possible after preparing it. Serving Size and Nutritional Information Calories: 273 per serving

net dietary fat 14.3 g Carbon dioxide: 29.4 g Carbohydrates: 35.7 g Carbon dioxide: 29.5 g

6.3 g of fiber

The following are the nutritional values for this dish: sugar (20 g); protein (4.8 g).

Sodium intake: 121 milligrams

Snack Recipes (Chapter 12):

Pumkin Seeds (Roasted)

Approximately 10 minutes are required for preparation. Approximately 20 minutes for preparation. 4 individual servings

Ingredients:

34 cup pumpkin seeds, soaked in water and then dried red chili powder (one-third teaspoon)

ground turmeric (14 teaspoon) depending on the situation

coconut oil (melted) (3 tablespoons)

Fresh lemon juice (approximately 12 tablespoons)

Directions:

350 degrees Fahrenheit (180 degrees Celsius) Preheat the oven.

Stir well to coat everything with oil and vinegar (except the lemon juice).

A baking sheet should be used to transfer the pumpkin seed mixture.

Turning once or twice during cooking time will ensure even browning.

Allow to cool completely before serving. Remove from oven and set aside.

Serve with a squeeze of fresh lemon juice. Calories and Nutritional Values per Serving There are 276 calories in a serving.

26.11 g (net) of total fat 4.9 g of carbohydrate 6.4 g of carbohydrate

Nutritional Values: 1.5 grams of fiber, 0.4grams of sugar, 8.6 grams of protein.

Amount of sodium in one serving: 69 mg

Almonds (Roasted)

Minutes required for preparation: 5 Approximately 10 minutes of preparation time 4 individual servings

Ingredients:

Whole almonds (about 1 cup total)

12-teaspoon cinnamon powder

ground cumin, 14 teaspoon

Season with salt and freshly ground black pepper to taste. olive oil (about 2 tbsp.

Directions:

Place parchment paper in the bottom of a baking dish.

Into a large mixing bowl, combine all of the ingredients and thoroughly combine.

A single layer of almonds should be spread out into a baking dish that has been prepared in advance of baking.

Turning twice during the roasting process.

Remove the almonds from the oven and set them aside to cool completely before serving them up.

Calories and Nutritional Values per Serving

Calories in a serving (198 calories)

18 g (net) of fat 2.2 g of carbohydrate 5.3 g of carbohydrate 3.1 g of fiber

The sugar content is one gram, and the protein content is four grams.

42 mg of sodium

The Cashews Are Sweet and Spicy!

Approximately 10 minutes are required for preparation. Approximately 20 minutes for preparation. Ingredients: 8 servings Nutritional Information:

cashews (about 2 cups)

2-tablespoons of unprocessed honey

A total of 12 teaspoons of smokey paprika

12 teaspoon red pepper flakes (optional). depending on the situation

lemon juice (about 1 tablespoon) olive oil (around 1 teaspoon)

Directions:

350 degrees Fahrenheit is the recommended temperature for the oven.

Place parchment paper in the bottom of a baking dish.

Stir together all of the ingredients in a large mixing basin until everything is well covered with sauce.

Using a single layer, transfer the cashew mixture to the baking dish that has been prepared.

Roast for 20 minutes, rotating about halfway through, until the potatoes are tender.

Allow to cool fully before serving. Remove from oven and put aside.

Calories and Nutritional Values per Serving

The following number of calories is 209:

16.5 grams of fat (net) 11.7 g of carbohydrate 12.9 g of carbohydrate

1.2 g of fiber

3.2 g of sucrose

5.3 g of protein

25 milligrams sodium

Chapter 10

Taco Chips (Tortillas)

15 minutes are required for preparation. Approximately 16 minutes for preparation. 6 portions (per serving)

The following are the ingredients: 112 cups shredded mozzarella cheese

tbsp of golden flaxseed meal 12 cup almond flour

Season with salt and freshly ground black pepper to taste.

375 degrees Fahrenheit is the temperature at which the oven should be preheated.

Put parchment paper on two baking sheets that are big enough to hold everything.

Cook for roughly 1 minute, stirring after every 15 seconds, in a microwave-safe dish, using cheese as a heat source.

Add the almond flour, flaxseed meal, salt, and black pepper to the bowl of melted cheese and stir thoroughly with a fork until everything is evenly distributed.

Knead the dough until it comes together in a ball.

The dough should be divided into two equally-sized balls.

Using a rolling pin, form each dough ball into an 8x10-inch rectangle on each baking sheet that has been prepped.

Make triangle-shaped chips out of each dough rectangle.

To make a single layer, arrange the chips.

Turn the pan halfway through and bake for another 10-15 minutes.

Remove the dish from the oven and leave it aside to cool before serving it to your guests.

Calories and Nutritional Values per Serving

Approximately 80 calories.

20.55 g (net) of fat 2. 5 g of carbohydrate 2.6 g of carbohydrate

The following nutrients are present: fiber (0.1 g), sugar (1.3 g), and protein (0.1 g).

6.3 g of protein

70 milligrams sodium

Beet Chips are a snack that is both healthy and delicious.

Approximately 10 minutes are required for preparation. Approximately 30 minutes of cooking time 4 individual servings

ingredients: thinly sliced beets, which have been cut, peeled, and cubed olive oil (around 1 tablespoon)

depending on the situation

Directions:

350 degrees Fahrenheit (180 degrees Celsius) Preheat the oven.

Place parchment paper on a baking pan and set aside.

Beet slices and oil should be combined in a large mixing basin and well mixed.

Prepare a baking sheet by arranging the beet slices in a single layer on the sheet.

30 minutes in the oven should enough. Calories and Nutritional Values per Serving Nutritional Values: 52 calories per serving

3.6 g (net) of total fat. There are four grams of carbohydrates in this recipe. 5 g of carbohydrate

1 gram of fiber

The sugar content is 4 g, while the protein content is 0.8g.

Amount of sodium in one serving: 77 mg

The combination of dates and oatmeal is a delicious combination. Cookies

15 minutes are required for preparation. Approximately 20 minutes for preparation. Ingredients: 8 servings Nutritional Information:

1/3 cup ground flaxseed (split into two halves) 6 tbsp. distilled water

Oats that cook quickly (about 1 cup) are used in this recipe.

old-fashioned oats (rolled): 1 cup tablespoon pumpkin pie spice (about a third of the cup)

12 teaspoon kosher salt (optional).

handmade pumpkin puree, melted coconut oil, and maple syrup 12 cups homemade pumpkin puree

Dates (about 12 cup), pitted and coarsely chopped

Directions:

350 degrees Fahrenheit is the recommended temperature for the oven.

A large baking sheet should be lined with parchment paper or silicone baking mats.

Stir together 2 tablespoons ground flaxseed and 1 cup water in a small mixing dish until thoroughly combined, about 30 seconds.

Remove from the oven and let aside for 10 minutes or so.

Combine the remaining ground flaxseed, oats, pumpkin seeds, pumpkin pie spice, and salt in a large mixing basin until thoroughly combined.

In a large mixing bowl, whisk together the pumpkin puree, flaxseed mixture, coconut oil, and honey until well incorporated.

Fold the date pieces in gently with your fingers. (Optional)

To bake, spread a single layer of the mixture onto the prepared cookie sheet and flatten each cookie slightly with your finger.

Prepare the oven for 15-20 minutes, or until the top is lightly browned.

Allow for about 5 minutes of cooling after removing the cookie sheet from the oven.

Invert the cookies onto a wire rack to allow them to cool completely before serving them.

Calories and Nutritional Values per Serving

Nutritious: 285 calories

15 g (net) fat 28.3 g of carbohydrates 33.4 g of carbohydrates

5.1 g of fiber

13 g of sucrose (sugar)

7 grams of protein

Amount of sodium in one serving: 125 mg

Croutons de Fromage

Time Required for Preparation: 20 min Approximately 14 minutes to prepare the dish 10 portions (per person).

Ingredients: 8 ounces cream cheese (or other soft cheese).

2 cups finely grated Parmesan cheese 1 cup finely grated Roman cheese Almond flour (one cup)

Egg (a single one).

dried rosemary (about 1 teaspoon)

Cajun seasoning (14 teaspoons) depending on the situation

Directions:

The oven should be set at 450 degrees Fahrenheit.

Place parchment paper on a baking pan and set aside.

Place the cream cheese, Parmesan cheese, Romano cheese, and almond flour in a microwave-safe bowl and microwave on "High" for approximately 1 minute, stirring once halfway through.

As soon as you remove it from microwave, whisk it vigorously until it is well blended.

Allow for about 2-3 minutes of cooling time.

Filling: In the same mixing bowl as the cheese, combine the egg, rosemary and seasonings with the salt until a dough forms.

Place the dough between two big parchment sheets on a flat surface and press down to flatten the dough.

Roll the dough out into a thin layer using a lightly floured rolling pin.

With a knife, cut the dough into desired-sized crackers after removing the top parchment paper sheet.

Prepare a baking sheet by arranging the crackers in a single layer, approximately 1 inch apart, on the prepared baking sheet.

Baking time is 6-7 minutes each side, or until the bacon is crispy.

Allow for thorough cooling after removing from the oven before serving.

Calories and Nutritional Values per Serving

Nutritional Values: 151 Calories

12.4 grams of fat (net) 1 gram of carbohydrate 2.7 g of carbohydrate

1.3 g of fiber

The amount of sugar in each serving is 0.4 g

9.8 g (of protein)

281 milligrams of sodium

Pizza with Sage and Walnuts (Chapter 13: Recipes for Pizza)

15 minutes are required for preparation. Approximately 20 minutes for preparation. 8 portions (per serving)

Ingredients:

frozen white bread dough, thawed 1 loaf frozen white bread dough, cut into 12-inch pieces 6 ounces Brie cheese, cut into 12-inch pieces 1 loaf frozen white bread dough

walnuts (chopped), 3 teaspoons

freshly chopped sage leaves (about 2 tablespoons total)

Directions:

400 degrees Fahrenheit is the recommended temperature for the oven.

Bake for 12 minutes at 400 degrees. Place the pizza dough on the baking sheet and roll out to a 12-inch diameter.

Press the edges together with your fingertips to create an outside border.

Indentations should be made into the dough using a fork.

Place the Brie cheese slices on top of the dough and sprinkle with the walnuts and sage, to finish.

Place the baking sheet in the oven for 20 minutes, or until the top begins to become golden.

Allow for around 5 minutes of cooling time after removing the pizza from the oven before slicing.

Then slice it up to your liking and serve it. Calories and Nutritional Values per Serving Nutritional Values: 356 calories

25.1% of total calories come from fat. 22.3 g of carbohydrate

24.55 g of carbohydrate

2.2 g of fiber

Sugar (0.2 g) is used in this recipe.

8.4 g (grams) protein

407 milligrams of sodium

Cooking Time: 15 minutes for the leeks and walnuts pizza

Approximately 25 minutes to prepare the dish 6 portions (per serving)

Ingredients:

Corn meal (about 1 tbsp. olive oil (around 1 teaspoon)

2 1/2 cups thinly sliced leek, if desired

frozen pizza dough (about 12 ounces)

134 cup grated Parmesan cheese 12 cup part-skim ricotta cheese 1/2 a clove of garlic, minced

salt (one-fourth teaspoon)

peppercorns (ground) (14 teaspoon) walnuts (about 2 teaspoons), finely chopped

Directions:

The oven should be set at 450 degrees Fahrenheit.

Cornmeal should be sprinkled over a baking sheet.

The leeks should be sautéed for around 10 minutes in a large nonstick wok over medium heat.

Set aside to cool after removing from the heat.

Placing the dough on a lightly floured board, roll it out into a 12-inch circle.

Place the rolled out dough on the baking sheet that has been prepared.

Press the edges together with your fingertips to create an outside border.

Mix the cheeses, garlic, salt, and black pepper in a large mixing basin until thoroughly combined.

Distribute the cheese mixture evenly over the pizza dough, leaving a 1-inch border around the edges.

Sprinkle walnuts on top of the leek mixture before serving.

Prepare the oven to bake for 15 minutes, or until the top is light golden.

Allow for around 5 minutes of cooling time after removing the pizza from the oven before slicing.

Then slice it up to your liking and serve it.

Calories and Nutritional Values per Serving

There are 371 calories in this recipe. Carbohydrates: 31.6g, 22.4g fat, 22.4g net fat 34.9 grams of carbohydrates 3.3 g of fiber

2.5 g of sucrose 8.6g of protein NaCl: 437 milligrams sodium An Onion that has been Caramelized Approximately 15 minutes to prepare the pizza. Approximately 25 minutes to prepare the dish Recipe serves 6 people; ingredients are as follows.

oil (olive) (two tablespoons)

2-cups onion, finely cut and split into rings. 1-pound pizza dough with an Italian cheese flavoring pizza sauce (12 cup) (bottled)

Sunflower seed oil (14 cup)

-drained and chopped sun-dried tomatoes; 1 cup crumbled goat cheese 3 ounces goat cheese

13/14 cup finely chopped fresh basil

Directions:

The oven should be set at 450 degrees Fahrenheit.

The onion should be cooked in the oil in a nonstick wok over medium-high heat when it has been heated through.

Allow 3-4 minutes of cooking time under cover.

Remove the lid and continue to boil for about 11 minutes, or until the potatoes are golden brown.

Using a baking sheet, place the pizza crust.

Add the pizza sauce and sun-dried tomatoes to a mixing bowl and combine well.

Top with the sautéed onion and cheese and then spread the sauce mixture over the top of the pizza dough.

For a golden brown crust, bake for 10 minutes or until the crust is crisp.

Remove the dish from the oven and sprinkle with fresh basil to finish it off.

Before slicing the pizza, let it alone for approximately 5 minutes.

Then slice it up to your liking and serve it.

Calories and Nutritional Values per Serving

There are around 300 calories in total. 9g (net) of fat There are 40.8 grams of carbohydrate in this recipe. 43.4 grams of carbohydrates 2.6 g of fiber

7.3 g of sugars 11.1g of protein 686 milligrams of sodium

CPSIA information can be obtained
at www.ICGtesting.com
Printed in the USA
BVHW011601200722
642495BV00014B/324